LIVING SAFELY, AGING WELL

LIVING SAFELY, AGING WELL

A Guide to Preventing Injuries at Home

DOROTHY A. DRAGO, M.P.H.

Johns Hopkins University Press
Baltimore

Note to readers

This book provides information to help older people and their spouses and children and other caregivers keep older people safe from injury. The information is as reliable and up-to-date as possible, but neither the author nor the publisher bears responsibility for the safety of an individual person. That responsibility lies with the person and with anyone providing care for that person.

This book is not intended to provide medical or legal advice. The services of a competent professional should be obtained whenever medical, legal, or other specific advice is needed. The publisher and the author make no warranty, either express or implied, regarding the recommendations offered or the practices described, nor does the publisher or the author assume liability for any consequences arising from the use of the content of this book.

© 2013 Johns Hopkins University Press
All rights reserved. Published 2013
Printed in the United States of America on acid-free paper
9 8 7 6 5 4 3 2 1

Johns Hopkins University Press
2715 North Charles Street
Baltimore, Maryland 21218-4363
www.press.jhu.edu

Library of Congress Cataloging-in-Publication Data

Drago, Dorothy A., 1946–
    Living safely, aging well : a guide to preventing injuries at home / Dorothy A. Drago, M.P.H.
        pages cm
    Includes bibliographical references and index.
    ISBN 978-1-4214-1151-4 (hardcover : alk. paper) — ISBN 978-1-4214-1152-1 (pbk. : alk. paper) — ISBN 1-4214-1151-2 (hardcover : alk. paper) — ISBN 1-4214-1152-0 (pbk. : alk. paper) — ISBN 1-4214-1153-9 — ISBN 978-1-4214-1153-8 (electronic)
    1. Older people—Health and hygiene. 2. Older people—Wounds and injuries—Prevention. 3. Accidents—Prevention. 4. Aging. 5. Self care, Health. I. Title.
    RA777.6.D73 2013
    613'.0438—dc23   2013010979

A catalog record for this book is available from the British Library.

With the following exceptions, all illustrations are by Loel Barr: Figures 1.1, 1.2, 1.3, and 1.4 are courtesy of the National Eye Institute.

Special discounts are available for bulk purchases of this book. For more information, please contact Special Sales at 410-516-6936 or specialsales@press.jhu.edu.

Johns Hopkins University Press uses environmentally friendly book materials, including recycled text paper that is composed of at least 30 percent post-consumer waste, whenever possible.

CONTENTS

LIVING SAFELY, AGING WELL

WHAT'S "OLD" GOT TO DO WITH IT?

Our definition of "old" changes over time. When we were children, we may have thought that 30 was old. In our thirties we probably thought that 50 was "over the hill." As we age, we push "old" into the future—to 65, say, the age long viewed by Social Security as normal retirement age. But as we approach 65, our concept of old age may drift to 75 or 80 or even older. Regardless of our personal perspectives on age, "old" today is older than it was a generation ago.

Part of the reason for this revised image of old age is that people are living longer. According to the U.S. Census Bureau, the population of Americans age 65 or older grew rapidly for most of the twentieth century, from 3.1 million in 1900 to 35.0 million in 2000. In April 2010, there were 40.3 million people 65 or older, constituting 13 percent of the total U.S. population. And the older population is on the threshold of a boom. The Census Bureau projects a substantial increase in the number of older people from 2010 to 2030; after all, the first Baby Boomers turned 65 in 2011. The older population in 2030 is projected to be twice as large as it was in 2000, growing from 35 million to 72 million. This group of people will represent nearly 20 percent of the U.S. population.

So, no matter how you define "old," there will soon be lots of old people—and these will be old people who will do what it takes to defend their independence and lifestyles. To maintain one's independence and lifestyle, however, one must age well; to age well, one must remain healthy; and to stay healthy, one must avoid injury. Whether you are an older person looking out for your own safety,

1

an adult child taking care of parents, or a caregiver helping someone stay safe from injury in the home, this book should provide much helpful—indeed critical—information.

If there were no increased risk of injury for older people compared to younger people, the rates of injury to people of different ages from the same cause would be the same, but they certainly are not. The U.S. Consumer Product Safety Commission has found that about three times as many adults 75 or older as one would expect are treated in hospital emergency rooms each year for injuries associated with consumer products. When older people are injured, their injuries are often more serious than a similar injury in a younger person, they may need to be hospitalized, they take longer to recuperate, they are at higher risk for infections and complications, and they are more vulnerable to repeat injuries. In short, people over age 75 are a fragile population when it comes to injuries. Since most accidents—including the majority among people 75 or older—happen at home, taking steps to be safe at home is essential.

What makes older persons so much more vulnerable to injury? While there is much individual variation in the aging process, age-related changes affect most older people. They include deterioration in the senses (vision, hearing, smell, taste, and touch) and an array of possible physical, cognitive, and health-related changes. Any of these alterations can make a person more susceptible to injury—whether it's the ability to recognize a hazard, the ability to react to it in time, or the greater likelihood of getting hurt than a younger person might under the same circumstances. Whether you are engaged in an everyday activity like walking or are using a harmless-seeming product like a vacuum cleaner or an obviously dangerous one like a car, your safety depends on the extent to which you have the abilities to meet the demands of the activity.

The rest of this chapter describes natural age-related changes and illustrates how they can contribute to increased risk of injury. No one can predict exactly when or to what degree these changes will begin to occur in any particular person. They may be so gradual that they aren't even noticed. Aging is highly personal! I will occasionally illustrate a point with examples from real life of people I have known.

PHYSICAL CHANGES

If we try to list the physical changes that go along with aging, we naturally think first of the most visible ones—wrinkles, graying hair, baldness, sagging skin, and so on—but these features are not important for safety. How safe a person is depends on how he or she functions in and interacts with the immediate environment—the activities and products involved in everyday life.

We spend our childhoods growing taller and stronger, and then most people plateau in height and strength as teenagers or young adults. Later, we realize that our youthful strength and stature do not endure. In general, people tend to get shorter and weaker as they age. These changes are related to natural alterations in bone and muscle structure. The amount of bone mass we have is greatest when we are about 30 years old; after that, bone loss continues faster than bone growth, resulting in ever-decreasing bone density. Loss of bone mass, called osteoporosis, is assumed to be one reason for the increase in bone fractures among older adults. It is also thought to be a factor in the flattening of the spinal vertebrae and the discs between them, as well as in the spontaneous fracture of vertebrae that some people experience—all of which contribute to making us shorter as we age. By some point between 65 and 79 years of age, most adults have lost about 3 to 6 percent of their peak height. At the same time that our bones are getting more fragile, our muscles are on the decline, too.

Men fare a bit better than women with regard to these particular physical changes. Men start with more bone and muscle mass than women do, and men do not go through menopause. Menopause brings reductions in hormones, like estrogen, and this contributes to bone loss in women.

The loss of bone and muscle mass can make it slower, more difficult, and sometimes painful to walk, get in and out of a chair, climb stairs, and do other simple physical activities. It can also affect fine motor skills, strength, and balance. These consequences of aging create a "fragile infrastructure" that makes it more challenging for us to function safely in our environment. It is therefore not surprising that bone and muscle deterioration are a major underlying cause of falls, which in turn are the most common cause of injury among older people. In addition, these physical changes increase older people's susceptibility to fractures, and if a fracture occurs before or as a result of a fall, the injury will take longer to heal. Fall-related injuries are the leading cause of death among people older than 75.

CHANGES IN THE SENSES

How accurately we see, hear, smell, taste, and feel diminishes with age. These changes in older people are not usually visible to others in the same way that loss of height and loss of muscle strength are, but there is other evidence that they are happening. For example, many people can't read small print when they get older. Or, an older person may often ask that someone repeat what they said, because they can't hear as clearly as they used to. Because we don't "see" these changes, we may forget that they are present, and we may not always be conscious of their impact on safety. Even the person experiencing sensory losses may not be conscious of their impact. Sensory impairment can decrease functional independence. In particular, reductions in hearing and vision can lead to isolation, depression, and withdrawal. The social impact of these losses is significant.

The effect of sensory losses on safety is enormous. When a person can't see clearly, she may take the wrong medication; when a person can't hear or smell well, he may not hear a teapot's whistle or smell the burning pot; when a person can't taste accurately, she may consume spoiled food and become ill; when a person has lost sensitivity in her hands, she may touch a hot surface but not remove the hand quickly enough to prevent a serious burn. By age 70, about one in five people have deficiencies in two senses, increasing their risk of injury and illness. People with both vision and hearing loss are more likely than those without either impairment to fall, break a hip, develop hypertension or heart disease, or have a stroke. Also important are two sensations not among the classic five senses, and those are sense of balance and sense of core body temperature.

Hearing

Hearing loss is the most common age-related sensory decline, affecting about one in three people aged 65 to 74, and nearly half of people 75 and older. Not only is reduced hearing the most common change, but it is the most gradual, making it difficult for the person to recognize and accept. Men are more likely than women to suffer hearing loss. Risk factors, in addition to aging, include smoking, a history of middle ear infections, exposure to certain ototoxic (damaging to the ear) chemicals or medications, head injury, tumors, stroke, and exposure to loud sounds. It is not unusual for construction workers, heavy equipment users, musicians, and military personnel to experience hearing loss.

Compared to other sensory deficiencies, hearing loss has the most damaging effect on social life. Not being able to hear well what people are saying to you or to share with others in activities that involve listening can lead to withdrawal, depression, and isolation. Observers may confuse hearing loss with dementia or forgetfulness, because the person who is missing much of what is being said may have trouble following a conversation. A person with hearing problems might even be mistaken as being uncooperative or nonresponsive.

In addition to its impact on social wellbeing, hearing loss puts people at increased risk for injury. They may not be able to hear a smoke alarm or a timer on the stove. They may not hear the phone ring or may answer the phone but not be able make out what is being said by the caller. Not hearing the siren or horn of a vehicle behind you while you are driving can be very dangerous. Any sound-generated alert or warning may be completely useless to a hearing-impaired person.

In spite of how deeply hearing loss impacts quality of life and personal safety, it is often undetected and untreated. Older people are less likely to have hearing evaluations and to use hearing aids than they are to have vision exams and to wear glasses. A partial explanation may be that there is still a stigma associated with wearing hearing aids, whereas glasses may be viewed as trendy and even attractive. (Hearing health care is addressed in detail in Chapter 9.)

Not all hearing loss is the same, and it isn't just sounds being softer than they used to be. Sometimes people lose the ability to recognize only certain kinds of sounds, like high-pitched sounds; sometimes speech seems mumbled; sometimes they can't distinguish between similar sounds; and hearing is often difficult when there is competing background noise, as there is in a loud restaurant. Some people with Alzheimer's disease or another kind of dementia effectively lose hearing ability, not because there is something wrong with their ears, but because their brain cannot interpret what the ears hear. The person can hear the sounds, but their brain cannot understand the meaning of the sounds. This situation causes additional confusion for them.

Hearing loss is usually gradual, with continuing degradation as people age; sometimes it can be sudden, the result of an infection, for example. Some people with hearing loss develop a ringing, hissing, or roaring sound in the ears; this condition is called tinnitus. The sounds may be intermittent or constant and may be soft or loud.

In communicating with older adults with impaired hearing, some people might employ "elderspeak," a simplified speech, with exaggerated intonation patterns, word stress, loudness, and speech timing. Elderspeak also uses simplified grammar, limited vocabulary, and a slow rate of delivery that is similar to the speech directed toward young children. The inclination to speak this way to people who seem to be having trouble hearing is understandable, but it can create unintended problems. While evidence indicates that elderspeak may improve older adults' comprehension, it also may contribute to giving them an "old" identity, reinforcing negative stereotypes about older adults, and lowering their self-esteem. Elderspeak can be viewed as patronizing. It can convey an impression of disrespect and a belief that the older person is cognitively and communicatively impaired. So, be cautious in using elderspeak if it seems called for; and if someone is using elderspeak in talking with you and you don't like it, say so.

Vision

After hearing loss, vision impairment and loss of visual acuity constitute the second most prevalent disability in people 65 or older.

Vision begins to decline earlier than any of the other senses do. Changes in some external parts of the eye, such as the cornea and lens, begin in a person's thirties or forties; changes to the retina (the tissue lining the inner surface of the eye) and to vision-related parts of the nervous system become noticeable in one's fifties and sixties. The greatest losses occur later in life. The near reading visual acuity of the average 70-year-old is 30 percent of that of a 20-year-old.

"Visual impairment" is defined as a vision loss that cannot be fully corrected by glasses or contact lenses alone. Underlying causes of visual impairment are cataracts, glaucoma, macular degeneration, and diabetic retinopathy.

Cataract describes a clouding of the lens of the eye; it makes the image the person sees fuzzy (as in Figure 1.1). Cataracts usually grow slowly, so the change in vision is gradual—the person may not notice it. Symptoms include blurry vision, seeing a "halo" around lights, perceiving headlights or other lights as being too bright at night, seeing colors as faded, and needing frequent changes in one's eyeglass prescription. Most cataracts are related to aging. Excess sun exposure and certain medications can stimulate or exacerbate cataract growth. Cataract-related loss of vision cannot be corrected with eyeglasses; surgery to replace the lens is required.

Glaucoma results in increased pressure in the eye. There is no pain along with the pressure, so a person may not realize that glaucoma is developing. Symptoms may include seeing things clearly in the center of the visual field but missing things in one's peripheral vision (see Figure 1.2). A person with glaucoma can end up with "tunnel vision." During an eye exam, when the optometrist or ophthalmologist sends that puff of air to your eye, he is measuring eye pressure, checking for signs of glaucoma.

Macular degeneration affects what a person sees in the middle of his visual field. The retina of the eye consists, in part, of specialized cells called rods and cones. The cones are for color vision, and the rods are for black-and-white vision. The macula is the central part of the retina. It is very rich in cones and it's where our vision is sharpest. There are two kinds of macular degeneration—dry and wet. Dry macular degeneration is more common, but we don't yet understand how or why it happens. Wet macular degeneration, which often leads to blindness, is caused when blood or another bodily fluid leaks behind the retina. Figure 1.3 shows what a person with macular degeneration might see.

Diabetic retinopathy is a form of damage to the blood vessels of the retina, caused by diabetes. The blood vessels may swell and leak fluid, or abnormal new blood vessels may grow on the surface of the retina. What a person with diabetic retinopathy sees is not only fuzzy but has blackened-out chunks in the visual field (see Figure 1.4). Diabetes also puts people at risk for developing cataracts and glaucoma at a younger age.

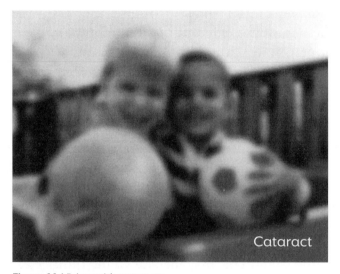

Figure 1.1. Vision with cataracts

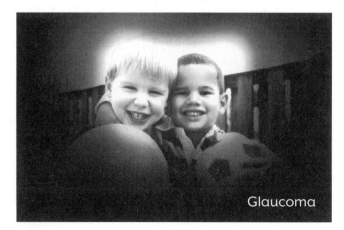

Figure 1.2. Vision with glaucoma

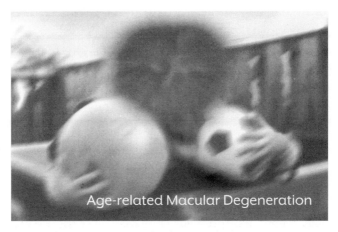

Figure 1.3. Vision with macular degeneration

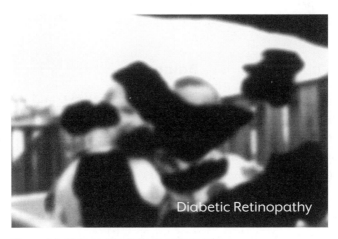

Figure 1.4. Vision with diabetic retinopathy

In people with Alzheimer's disease or another kind of dementia, the same functional disability can happen with their vision as happens with their hearing. That is, how well they can see things declines, not because there is something wrong with their eyes, but because their brain cannot understand or interpret the messages the eye is collecting and sending to the brain. I observed this in my mother, and at the time I thought maybe she just needed new eyeglasses. I remember her being seated at the dinner table but not "seeing" the fork she was to eat with. When I had told her several times where the fork was and she still asked, "Where?" I realized that her brain had lost the ability to understand the signal sent from her eyes conveying the image of the fork.

The inability to see our surroundings clearly increases our risk of injury. For example, we might take the wrong medicine if the bottles appear similar, or take the wrong amount if we cannot read or understand the label; we might trip and fall if we cannot see obstructions in our path or if we have poor depth perception; and we might incorrectly adjust a heating pad too high and be at risk for burns.

As can happen to people with hearing loss, some people with diminished vision begin to withdraw because they feel uncomfortable in their surroundings. They may choose not to go out, insecure because they can't get around well. They may alter their gait, adopting a more cautious way of walking. Feeling at risk may make them limit what they do, which in turn can affect their social and other activities, and lead to depression.

Balance

Poor physical balance increases the risk of falling, and it is related to the two sensory losses just described. Vision and hearing are two of the senses that work together to help us know where we are in space; we see our surroundings and hear sounds, and the vestibular system (the balance system that works in concert with the hearing system) tells us where our head is in space, keeping us upright and not dizzy. Losses in vision and hearing, and disruptions to the vestibular system can put us out of touch with our environment. Not knowing where we are in space can affect our sense of balance.

Besides being affected by vision and hearing loss, the ability to keep our balance can also be affected by poor nutrition, reactions to certain medications, low blood pressure, low blood sugar, vertigo, light-headedness, and reduced muscular strength, to name a few factors. Age-related changes in the vestibular system can begin before age 30; by age 70, there can be as much as a 40 percent decline in the number of vestibular nerve and inner ear hair cells, which are very important to balance. This decline can make it difficult for older persons to determine if they are moving in space or if it is the world that is moving around them. Feeling off balance or dizzy, feeling as if you are spinning, or not having a clear sense of where your head and body are in space all make it harder to avoid falls and collisions with objects.

Smell and Taste

Smell and taste are related senses in that what we taste is influenced by what we smell. Age takes a greater toll on smell than on taste. Sense of smell begins to diminish around age 60. During the aging process, the number of taste buds we have actually decreases, and the remaining ones get smaller. At around age 75, we have only about a third of the taste buds we had at 30. With a poorer sense of smell, people are deprived of early warnings that most of us take for granted. Smell alerts us to fires, poisonous fumes, and gas leaks; taste warns us of spoiled food and drink and of substances that are inappropriate for eating. A 2008 study found that people who had lost their sense of smell or had an impaired sense of smell were significantly more likely than those with a normal sense of smell to burn food when cooking and to eat spoiled food. And, of course, they were less likely to detect a gas leak and to smell a fire.

Decreases in sense of smell and taste lead many people to eat less or to eat less nutritious food. For most of us, food is a source of pleasure as well as of nutrition, and when the pleasure diminishes, there is less motivation to eat. Like vision and hearing losses, loss of smell and taste can lead to reduction of social activity and to depression.

Touch and Core Temperature

When my elderly father was living with me, I often would get upset with him for having dirty or sticky fingers and leaving hand prints on the fridge and table tops. Only much later did I realize that he had lost much of the feeling in his fingertips due to a combination of chronic disease and aging. Loss of sensation in extremities can be associated with diabetes (which my father had), poor circulation, or neurological problems. Even if a person does not have a chronic illness, with aging comes a reduction in the ability of the skin to discriminate the pressure and vibration associated with touch.

Aside from personal hygiene issues, loss of sensation of touch can also increase the risk of injury. For example, not being able to feel the sharp edge of a knife can lead to cuts, and not realizing when something hot is too hot can result in scalds and thermal burns (scalds involve a hot liquid or steam; thermal burns involve a hot surface). The comfort of appropriately warm bath water or a heating pad can turn into a scald or thermal burn hazard if excessively hot temperatures go unnoticed.

In addition to a reduced sense of feeling in extremities, older people's sensation of their core temperature can become less accurate, because of, among other factors, skin-related changes. Maintaining overall normal body temperature is critical to survival. Being too hot (hyperthermia) or too cold (hypothermia) can be very serious and even cause death. Most of us have heard that older people are more susceptible than younger people to illness and death from heat waves and from winter cold.

COGNITIVE CHANGES

The speed and the processes of cognition—how we know and learn things—change as we get older. As we age, certain parts of our brains shrink—the parts important to learning, memory, planning, and other complex mental activities. The typical cognitive functions affected by age are memory and attention. Most of us will experience some degree of forgetfulness. Where are those keys? Who was that person? What's the word I'm looking for? What did you tell me to bring? All of these examples of memory loss are a normal part of aging. While there is much variation among individuals, and while some adults retain excellent cognitive function well into their seventies and eighties, on average, people have begun to experience some minimal decline in cognitive abilities by their middle to late sixties and a more pronounced decline after age 75.

The high-tech world we live in today presents a good example of this cognitive slowing. Every day most of us deal with automatic teller machines (ATMs), microwave ovens, smart phones (which seem to do everything else in addition to allowing conversation between individuals), computers, cable boxes, remote controls, and more. Typically, when an older person has trouble with one of these products, the first person consulted is someone much younger—for many reasons: younger people grew up with these products, they are highly flexible cognitively, and their minds work in synch with how the products work, that is, they think like the products work. In contrast, older people's brains cannot process as quickly the information necessary to carry out sequences of steps, like the series and combinations of buttons to press in order to complete tasks on electronic products. When receiving instruction on these products, the older person may not be able to keep his attention focused long enough to learn what to do. They may have to "look longer" at something in order to understand, because older brains simply aren't as nimble as young brains. Because tasks can take longer to finish and the person may make errors along the way, he or she may give up in frustration.

Dementia is different from the cognitive lapses of normal aging and can have one or more of several causes. It is not a disease but rather a group of symptoms that can include impaired judgment, increasing difficulty in finding words, mood or personality changes, and difficulty remembering how to do familiar activities. According to the National Institute on Aging, about one in seven people aged 71 or over has dementia. The most common cause of dementia in older people is Alzheimer's disease, a neurodegenerative disease that encompasses more than just memory loss. Another cause is stroke. Alzheimer's disease affects 5 to 10 percent of people over age 65 and 20 to 40 percent of individuals over age 80. The distinction between Alzheimer's disease and other types of dementia is not important for the purposes of this book. What is important is that any loss of cognitive function, regardless of the underlying cause, can increase the risk of injury.

SEEING THE WHOLE PICTURE

The age-related changes described above usually come on gradually. Eventually, most people who live beyond age 60 will be experiencing a few of them simultaneously. In addition, individuals may have other health-related challenges, such a low blood pressure, diabetes, or heart disease, that impact everyday life and safety.

It's not as if an aging person has just one issue at a time to deal with. Here's an example from my own experience. I came home one evening and smelled burning rubber in the house. I tracked the scent to the kitchen sink mat, but I was perplexed as to how it had been burned. The next day, I found out what happened. Over break-fast, my 90-year-old dad explained. He had put a pot of prunes on the stove to cook and gone into another room to watch TV. At some point, all the water boiled off the prunes, and the pan itself began cooking. I don't know if my father had set the stove timer—he had had trouble learning how to do that. If he had, he probably would not have heard it in any case; because of his hearing loss, he always had the TV blaring. I don't know if the smoke alarm went off; he might not have heard it for the same reason. The pan was damaged enough that he should have smelled something out of the ordinary, but he hadn't. When he realized what was happening, he took the hot pot directly from the stove and placed it in the sink. That was a reasonable course of action, but he apparently didn't process or detect the consequences of placing the burning pan on the rubber mat. Here was an example of multiple age-related sensory deprivations (hearing, smelling, and cognition) synergistically interacting to put a person at risk for a house fire.

The various changes associated with aging can combine to exaggerate the effect of each one singly. The more areas where there are losses, the more a person is put at risk for injury.

Injuries are not random events, and that's why understanding injury prevention and home safety for older adults can help you have a little more control over dangerous events. There are always circumstances that "set the stage" for injury. The stage includes the person, a thing (which I will call a product) being used by the person, and the use environment. Each of these factors can contribute to or be a direct cause of an injury. Let me give you another example. An 82-year-old who has some dementia (the person) is trying to heat water for tea on a stove (the product) in her kitchen (the environment). She is wearing a robe (another product) with long, loose sleeves. She reaches to the back of the stove to turn the knob for a rear burner, but instead, she gets confused and turns on a front burner—the one her arm is reaching over. Her sleeve catches fire, and she doesn't know what to do. She is seriously burned before anyone realizes what has happened.

What might have created a different outcome in this scenario? (1) If someone, for example a relative or friend of the person, knew of her tendency to get confused about the knobs on the stove, that person could have marked one knob with a color, and this knob would be *the only knob the woman was allowed to touch*; or the stove could have been made impossible for the woman to use by covering the knobs with a device used to keep young children from operating knobs. (2) The designer of the stove could have put the knobs in a less hazardous location that would have avoided anyone's having to reach over the burners. This could have been considered when the stove was purchased. (3) If someone assisted the woman in dressing, or if someone monitored her wardrobe, she could have been dressed in a garment with tighter-fitting sleeves that would not have dipped so close to the open flame and caused such rapid flame spread.

When you anticipate the possibility of an injury, you can attempt to prevent it. The point of this book is to help you understand aging as a risk factor for injury, help you recognize circumstances that put older people at risk for injury, and explain what you can do to help yourself or someone else avoid injury. I'm not saying it will always be simple or easy, but I am saying you can make a difference in potential outcomes. Many older people want their surroundings to remain unchanged. If someone else suggests removing a rug that is a tripping hazard, the response might be, "Don't you dare take away that rug—I love that rug." Ideally, older persons and the people who care about them, working collaboratively, can improve their safety without conflict. Perhaps the rug could be hung on the wall, like a tapestry, or put to use in some other fashion.

There will be challenges. If you are an adult child or friend trying to make an older person safer, there will be successes and there will be failures. We are all human. We do the best we can. But, because injuries in older age can be so life altering, it is worth trying hard to prevent them.

As you read the following chapters in this book, you will see that many aspects of one's life affect the risk of injury. The most promising way to stay safe from injury is to adopt a "lifestyle" approach. While I make specific recommendations to improve household safety, you will see that lifestyle choices have the deepest effect on safety. Staying injury free means taking care of the whole person: exercising; eating well; taking care of your illnesses and diseases; seeing your doctor; attending to vision and hearing losses; engaging in intellectually stimulating activities; keeping strong social ties to family, friends, and community; believing that preventive measures work; and putting them into practice.

2

DON'T FALL!

When an older person falls, there is, unfortunately, a good chance that the person's quality of life will be severely diminished. Whether as the result of an injury suffered in the fall, an increased fear of falling, or reduced confidence in the ability to perform daily tasks, many older people lose some or even most of their independence after a fall. Sometimes people are lucky and suffer no injury or only a minor injury in a fall, but often enough falls result in broken bones and hospitalizations. And some falls cause fatal injuries.

These figures will give you an idea of the magnitude of the problem: In 2010 in the United States, more than half a million people aged 65 to 74 years were injured in a fall and about a million and a half people 75 or older were injured as a result of a fall. In 2009, nearly three thousand people aged 65 to 74 years and more than seventeen thousand people aged 75 or older died as a result of a fall.

No matter what sources you consult, they all draw the same conclusion: falls are the primary injury mechanism for the aging population. These sources also say that if a person falls once, the likelihood of a second fall is nearly doubled and that the risk of being seriously injured in a fall increases with age. This doesn't mean that falls are a normal part of aging and that they are inevitable. To the contrary, risk factors for falling vary among individuals. For this reason, a person's individual risks can be identified, and then appropriate strategies to address those particular risks can be put in place.

The U.S. Consumer Product Safety Commission (CPSC) collects data on consumer product related injuries. The CPSC defines consumer products as those used in and around the home, in schools, and in recreation. More than half (59%) of consumer product–related emergency room visits for adults 65 to 74 years of age involve falls; 77 percent of consumer product–related emergency room visits for adults aged 75 or older involve falls. Typical fall scenarios include falling down stairs; falling out of bed; tripping over rugs, cords, or other obstacles on the floor; and falling off ladders and step stools.

Here are some other facts about falls:

- More falls happen in the home than anywhere else.

- Women are more likely to fall, but men are more likely to die from a fall.

- After a fall, some people develop a fear of falling again. This fear can cause people to limit their activities, leading to reduced mobility and physical fitness, and thus, ironically, increasing their risk of falling.

Knowing that falls are a common source of injury is not as helpful as knowing *why* people fall. Knowing *why* allows us to do something about it. There is no single or simple way to explain why people fall, however. Usually, there are multiple reasons for a fall. Remember that we humans are complicated and complex, and we interact with numerous environments. During most human activities, a lot is going on at the same time, and there are many factors that affect the chances of falling—what safety experts call fall risk factors.

Fall risk factors can be grouped into two broad categories: internal (or intrinsic) factors—those within the person; and external (or extrinsic) factors—those outside the person. Figures 2.1 and 2.2 identify some internal and external fall risk factors. Separating risk factors into these two categories is a very good way to understand which factors we have control over and can change and which factors we don't have good control over and may find hard to change.

It may seem that factors inside ourselves would be easier to address and modify than those outside ourselves. However, ironically, internal risk factors are more difficult to change than external ones, and unfortunately the intrinsic factors may have more significant impact on risk of falling than extrinsic ones do. According to current research, the strongest risk factors for falls include: previous falls; strength, gait, and balance impairments; and medications—all intrinsic factors. Some additional intrinsic fall risk factors are: the

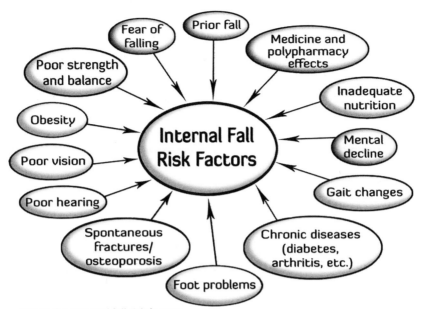

Figure 2.1. Internal fall risk factors

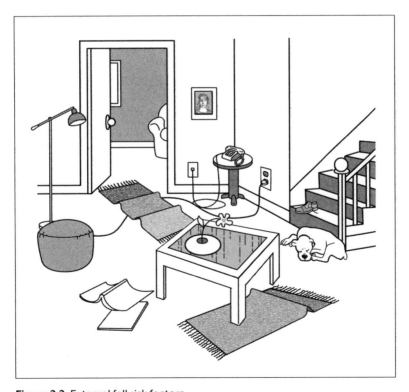

Figure 2.2. External fall risk factors

presence of illness or disease, nutritional status, degradation in the function of the senses (especially vision and hearing), foot conditions, fear of falling, and mental decline. Obviously, intrinsic factors vary from individual to individual. So, the first question to ask is, "What are the specific fall risk factors intrinsic to this person?" and the second question is, "How can these intrinsic fall risk factors be reduced?"

INTRINSIC FALL RISK FACTORS

In the following sections, I discuss all the intrinsic factors that the published scientific literature supports as being contributing factors to falls. Some factors may jump right off the page as being very relevant to you; others may not seem relevant at all.

Since having fallen once is a significant risk factor for falling again, preventing that first fall is doubly important. Here are the key means of counteracting internal fall risk factors when trying to prevent a first fall:

✓ Keep physically strong.

✓ Eat well to ensure good nutrition.

✓ Know what medicines you are taking and be aware of side effects.

✓ Have your vision and hearing tested regularly.

✓ Have foot problems checked by a podiatrist.

Let's take these prevention strategies one at a time and consider how they relate to falls and falls prevention.

Strength, Balance, and Gait

A person's overall physical condition is a contributing factor in falls. As noted in Chapter 1, most people lose muscle and bone mass as they age, which means they lose physical strength, too. Strength is needed to move your body, like getting up from a chair, and to maintain balance. An important consequence of decreased strength is that people may change their activity level, from active, to moderately active, to sedentary. Reducing activity creates a circle of decline: the less active people are, the more strength they lose, and then in turn they become even less active. Decreased physical activity translates to decreased muscle mass, strength, and power. So, staying strong is crucial to preventing falls. (It has countless other benefits, as well.)

Research has shown that physical strength and balance can be improved through exercise. When improved and maintained, strength and balance become fall protective factors. Many fall prevention programs include exercise (strength training, balance, stretching, and so on) to help with physical fitness. The 2011 American Geriatric Society Guidelines recommend that all fall prevention programs include an exercise component. The greatest positive effects of exercise on fall rates were seen in programs that included a combination of a high total dose of exercise and challenging balance exercises. Interestingly, these programs did *not* include walking, probably because walking itself can be a risk for falling, as you will read later on in this chapter. (This does not mean that if you walk for exercise and are comfortable doing so you should stop.) Some programs involve tai chi or yoga, including yoga done while seated in a chair. These practices help improve balance and strength, and for some offer the added benefit of feeling calm and grounded. A 2012 study added another dimension to the fall prevention role of exercise. The findings of the study suggest that exercise reduces the chance of falls because it improves cognitive function, especially so-called executive functions like planning, working memory, attention, problem solving, verbal reasoning, appropriate inhibition, mental flexibility, and multitasking.

Decide with your doctor what kinds of exercises are appropriate for you, then choose a program you think you might enjoy. For many people, exercising on their own is neither fun nor motivational. Such persons should look for exercise programs offered at community centers, gyms, councils on aging, hospitals, and so on. You may be surprised at the variety of classes available. With a class, there is the added benefit of social interactions, which help keep a person mentally healthy. Some people prefer not to exercise with a group. They may choose to exercise at a gym but not in a class;

personal trainers are usually available for a fee, or they may offer a complimentary, one-time consultation to sketch out a strength and balance regimen for an individual. Many people make a pact with a friend to exercise together.

A new exercise approach is described as exergaming—a combination of video gaming and exercise. Could this combination be for you? Apparently, the enjoyable and challenging nature of video game–based exercising motivates people to exercise. A study from the Netherlands showed that persons who engaged in exergaming experienced improved balance as well as improved task performance.

Because more than half of the falls that occur while a person is walking involve tripping, gait and balance are critical intrinsic factors in avoiding falling. (The obstacle that one trips on is an extrinsic risk factor.) Gait is simply the way we walk—how our feet touch and then lift off the floor. Balance is control over one's center of gravity. Gait and balance, although separate entities, are often intertwined. For example, changes in bone structure that accompany osteoporosis often result in curvature of the spine. When the spine is curved, the head tends to be positioned forward relative to the rest of the body. Having the head positioned more forward instead of in line with the body alters the person's center of gravity and can throw the person off balance, which in turn can lead to a change in gait. The head is pretty heavy! Imagine carrying a bowling ball out in front of you for any length of time, and you can appreciate that you would have to change your gait to compensate for the resulting change in your center of gravity. Thus, a change in gait can often be an important symptom that a person's health status has changed.

We may take balance for granted, but it is very complex. The upright body is basically unstable and relies on perceptions of its surroundings to maintain balance. Those perceptions include what we see around us, what the vestibular system in our inner ear tells us about where we are in space, and what our feet tell us about the kind of surface beneath us. All of that information has to be processed cognitively so that the brain can tell the body how to maintain balance. And finally, the muscles have to be able to move the body to make the necessary adjustments to stay balanced.

Think of walking as a continuous process of losing and regaining balance. At some point in every gait cycle, one foot pushes off the ground and moves through the air before it comes down again, usually heel first. While that foot was in the air, the weight was on the other foot. Most falls occur at the moment when the weight is being transferred from one foot to the other—that is, when the toes of the back foot and the heel of the front foot are in contact with the ground.

The published scientific literature confirms that gait changes are common among older persons and that they contribute to the risk of tripping and falling. Here are some examples of abnormal types of gaits: cautious, weak, fear-of-falling, freezing (feet feel glued to the ground but the body moves forward), and *marche à petit pas* (taking small steps). The most significant and observable age-related change in gait is slowed walking speed, primarily related to a shorter stride length. Other types of age-related gait change are a more flat-footed contact with the ground, a toed-out stance, or not lifting the feet as high off the ground while walking. The underlying causes of gait changes are many; they include, but are not limited to, a painful or disfiguring foot condition, a fear of falling, a prior stroke, loss of strength, neurological changes, and reduced range of motion in the ankle joint.

To assess a person's gait, observe how he walks; to assess your own gait, have someone watch while you walk. These are the questions the observer should ask:

- Does he take full steps, placing the heel down first?

- Does he shuffle?

- Does he walk slowly or quickly?

- Does he have good balance?

I can recall how my mother's gait changed from what I would consider a normal gait to a shuffle, her feet barely lifting off the floor. Her gait change was related to her dementia. With this change, her interaction with carpeting and thresholds was suddenly different and more hazardous. A gait change can make a person more prone to tripping; being aware of such a change can motivate you to make environmental (extrinsic) changes to reduce the risk of falls.

Nutrition

A factor related to strength—and therefore to risk of falling—is nutrition. While we need fewer calories per day as we age, we still need good nutrition. There are six categories of nutrients that the body needs to acquire from food: protein, carbohydrates, fat, fibers, vitamins and minerals, and water. Do not underestimate the need for water! Water is necessary for metabolism, excretion, and assimilation of nutrients. Dehydration is dangerous. It can make a person dizzy or disoriented and can cause muscle cramping. General guidelines for good nutrition tell us to eat a variety of foods, including plenty of vegetables, fruits, and whole grain products; to eat lean meats, poultry, fish, beans, and low-fat dairy products; and to keep salt, sugar, alcohol, and fat intake modest.

Vitamin D supplements are often recommended for older persons as a way to address bone loss. Among its several benefits, vitamin D seems to play a role in fall prevention, with the strongest benefit being for older men. Studies have shown that a low vitamin D level in the blood was associated with disturbed gait control. Other studies have shown that vitamin D supplements are effective only in people who are deficient in vitamin D to begin with.

Another nutritional component associated with fall prevention is folate. One study which investigated vitamin D, folate, and vitamin B12 showed that serum (blood) levels of folate were significantly lower in people who were prone to falling.

Before you run out and buy dietary supplements of these or any other compounds, remember that taking supplements cannot replace a balanced diet, and taking supplements can be dangerous. Pills usually concentrate the amount of a substance. As an example, vitamin E supplements contain anywhere from 100 to 1,000 IU (international units) per pill. Consider that you would have to eat *four cups of almonds* (rich in vitamin E) to get 100 IU of vitamin E. Also consider that the daily recommended dose of vitamin E for adults is only 22.4 IU. Consult your doctor about taking supplements—whether you should take them, and if so, which ones, how much, and how often.

Medications

Many older people take medication to treat high blood pressure, high cholesterol, depression, diabetes, arthritis, and a host of other problems. In fact, the average older American may be taking four different prescription medications at the same time. Some of these medicines have side effects—perhaps nausea, dizziness, or constipation, for example. The more medications we take, the greater are the chances of unwanted side effects. If side effects occur, we may be given additional medications to take to address the adverse reactions of the other medications. The result is called polypharmacy, the taking of multiple drugs at the same time when some of them are to counter adverse effects of other medications being taken. A recent study reported that polypharmacy can be more of a fall risk factor than the diseases for which the original medicines were prescribed.

The following is a hypothetical example of how polypharmacy can increase the risk of falling. Bill takes a prescription drug that causes him some nausea and gastric irritation. To address the nausea and gastric irritation, he takes an additional drug, which in turn causes him to retain fluid. He takes a pill to help eliminate the fluid, but that pill causes dizziness. To address the dizziness, he takes another medication. Bill started taking one drug and ended up taking four. Consider that Bill's fluid pill causes him to urinate with greater frequency, including needing to get up during the night. If he experiences dizziness, and is walking to the bathroom in the middle of the night (most likely in low light, and without his glasses), he has greatly increased his chances for a fall.

Some medications raise particular concerns for falls, and thus it is important that someone monitor people who are taking that medication. These drugs include blood pressure medications, medicines for diabetes, and anti-anxiety medications—all of which have the potential to cause dizziness. Neither very high nor very low blood pressure is good. Low blood pressure or a sudden drop in blood pressure can make you dizzy and unsteady on your feet, and thus increase the likelihood of a fall. While high blood pressure in itself usually has no symptoms, treatment of high blood pressure can make you dizzy. A recent study conducted in England found that thiazide antihypertensive drugs (those that reduce blood pressure by increasing urine output) were associated with an increased risk of falls, especially in the first three weeks of taking them. Although the researchers did not mention getting up in the middle of the night to urinate as a possible factor, another study noted that many falls occur between midnight and 6 a.m. Another study recommended that fall prevention programs include an assessment of the person's urination frequency and referral for treatment to ease symptoms of urge incontinence.

Treatment of diabetes requires monitoring of blood sugar. If blood sugar is too high, adjustment to diet or medication is necessary. If blood sugar drops too low (called hypoglycemia), a person can become dizzy and unsteady and thus be at increased risk for a fall. Therapeutic insulin, a hormone given to people who have diabetes to lower their blood sugar, has been shown to be a risk factor for falls among older persons. This suggests a relationship between the treatment and its potential to result in too low a level of blood sugar, and it emphasizes the importance of closely monitoring a patient on this medication. So, persons with diabetes are well advised to accurately track their blood sugar and take measures to improve their safety, since both the disease and certain treatments are risk factors for falling.

Anti-anxiety drugs are commonly prescribed for older people who show signs of agitation. There is a high incidence of dizziness as a side effect from these medications. A Canadian study that examined falls in an older population for whom an anti-anxiety medication had been prescribed (most commonly lorazepam or zopiclone) found that among patients who fell, nearly half had begun taking the anti-anxiety medication within seven days before the fall.

These are only a few kinds of medications that are associated with an increased risk for falls. Others can pose the same risk. All medications should be taken exactly as directed, that is, the correct amount at the recommended times of day for the number of days indicated, and the patient should be monitored for possible medication-related changes. Many older people are on medications for lengthy periods of time, some perhaps for the rest of their lives.

It is good practice to periodically review with your doctor and/or pharmacist all the medicines you are taking, so any potential fall risks can be brought to light. Another reason to review medications is to identify any potential drug interactions and identify any potential for overdosing by taking multiple medications that contain the same active ingredients. Be sure to review over-the-counter (OTC) nonprescription drugs, including herbal preparations and supplements. Because OTC medications are convenient, relatively inexpensive, widely available, and don't require a prescription, people may view them differently from prescription drugs and may treat them as if they could be taken liberally, without concern, and without side effects. But OTC medicines also have a maximum daily dosage, a limited overall period for taking the medicine, and specific instructions—for example to take the medicine with food—and these admonitions should be adhered to with the same care you would take with a prescription drug.

A study based on a review of the literature from 1966 through 2008 showed an increased risk for falls in older individuals exposed to NSAIDs (nonsteroidal anti-inflammatory drugs), although it did not elaborate on the reasons. Some common over-the-counter NSAIDs are aspirin, ibuprofen (Advil and Motrin), and naproxen (Aleve). These drugs are popular among the older population because they ease arthritis pain and are generally perceived as being safe (although taken in excess they can cause stomach problems, including ulcers).

Finding a balance between taking the drugs that are necessary for one's health and comfort and avoiding injury related to polypharmacy will be one of the biggest challenges for public health professionals in this century. Doctors and patients need to work together to monitor how many and which drugs and remedies are being taken. The goal is not to find a set number of medications and try to stay below that number but to find the right medications at the right dosages and for the shortest possible duration. Tell your doctor these are the criteria you want followed when your medications are prescribed. This approach may keep your treatment safer and more effective and may also help improve your quality of life. (Medicine related poisoning is discussed in Chapter 3.)

Vision and Hearing

Seeing clearly, including having good depth perception, is extremely important for fall prevention. It has been reported that people with reduced visual acuity are 1.7 times more likely to fall and 1.9 times more likely to have multiple falls compared to fully sighted people. Regular eye exams are recommended especially as we age, not only to ensure adequate magnification, but also as a way to detect cataracts, glaucoma, macular degeneration, and other serious eye problems early in their development. Many people 65 or older do not get regular eye exams because they believe there is no need, but vision is very much a factor in good overall health. Perhaps because poor vision does not make one "sick" in the traditional sense, it may not be taken as seriously as a condition that has a more obvious or a painful physical effect.

While eyeglasses are a helpful aid, changes in magnification can, ironically, increase the risk of falls *in the short term*. You may have had the experience of an adjustment period after your glasses prescription has been changed. But don't let this keep you from addressing your future vision needs; you just need to be aware of how changes in magnification can affect your gait and make you more susceptible to falls while you are getting used to the prescription. If your new prescription makes things bigger, they appear closer; if it makes things smaller, they appear more distant. These differences in depth perception can affect our movements. We may think we have placed a foot on a step or curb before we actually reach that step or curb. We may take higher, shorter steps. These are natural gait adjustments in response to changes in magnification. Getting used to new glasses requires a bit of time, but our eyes and brains do adjust reasonably quickly. It is much safer in the long run to have corrected vision.

Have you ever had an eyeglass prescription that was "off"? Did it make you dizzy or affect your balance? If a person experiences any dizziness or problems seeing clearly after a new prescription, he should go back to the optometrist or ophthalmologist and have the prescription rechecked. Dizziness that cannot otherwise be medically explained might be due, for example, to a bifocal lens sitting too high in the eyeglasses and interfering with distance vision.

While a person may not detect the problem, the person's body may react by losing its sense of balance. Remember, what we see helps orient us in space.

More serious eye impairments, like cataracts and macular degeneration, contribute to falls because they can reduce contrast sensitivity and visual clarity (see Chapter 1). Early cataract surgery has been shown to reduce the rate of falls.

A secondary effect of vision problems is that people may decide to become less mobile. When people do not move, they lose muscle strength. Thus, one impairment—reduced vision—affects a totally different fall risk factor—strength. We begin to see how a combination of factors can make matters even worse. One study showed that poor vision itself was not as significant a factor in falls as the fact that the low vision made the person less active. The loss of strength from inactivity was the greater risk factor.

Hearing loss may not be as obvious a risk factor for falling as vision loss, but it nonetheless is a factor, in part because of its close relationship to balance. With hearing loss, we can lose some sense of where we are in space—and that loss affects a person's sense of balance, increasing the risk of falls. A hearing problem can be indicative of an underlying balance problem, and a balance problem can be indicative of an underlying hearing loss, so pursuing good hearing health is indeed a part of maintaining overall good health in addition to being a fall prevention measure. A 2012 study found that having a hearing loss, regardless of whether it is moderate or severe, triples the risk of falling for people in their forties and older.

Vision and hearing health care are addressed in Chapter 9.

Feet

There is increasing evidence that foot problems and inappropriate footwear increase the risk of falls. Non-healing foot sores, foot deformity, pain associated with deep calluses, and not clipping one's toenails have all been associated with falls. Certain disease conditions, for example diabetes, can affect the feet and have a significant effect on fall risk. A condition called diabetic neuropathy (which is diabetes-related nerve damage) can cause numbness in the feet, which in turn makes it very difficult for the feet to "sense" where they are in space and to respond appropriately when contacting surfaces. We may not realize how much important information we sense through our feet, such as where the edge of a step is or whether we are walking on level or sloping ground.

Taking good care of one's feet and toenails may become more difficult as we get older. We may not be able to easily reach our feet because of reduced flexibility; we may not see clearly enough to perform the cutting and cleaning of toenails; arthritis may reduce the strength or dexterity of our hands, making using nail clippers or scissors difficult. People who have diabetes may not be able to feel what they are doing, and as a result they may do more harm than good. Poor foot care can result in pain and infection. Seeing a podiatrist can often be beneficial. (See Chapter 9.) Given all that our feet do for us, they deserve to be well cared for.

Summary of Steps to Reduce Intrinsic Fall Risk Factors

Keep physically active, within what's reasonable, to help maintain strength. Consider an exercise program that includes balance practice. Many gyms and councils on aging offer programs tailored for the older population. Yoga and tai chi are also popular and are excellent for this age group.

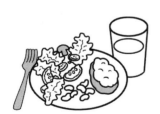

Eat a balanced diet and drink plenty of water. Pay attention to any diet restrictions the doctor has ordered. Have someone help with food shopping and preparation if necessary.

Routinely have your vision and hearing checked, as these senses affect balance.

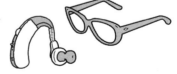

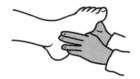

Take good care of your feet. See a podiatrist as needed.

Know what medicines you are taking and
make note of any side effects you experience. Review your medication history,
both prescription and over-the-counter,
with your doctors and other health providers.

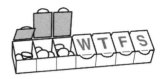

EXTRINSIC FALL RISK FACTORS

Let's now turn to extrinsic risk factors for falls. Extrinsic factors are
those "outside" the person. Here are examples of extrinsic factors:
clothing and shoes the person wears; any walking aids, like canes,
crutches, and walkers; and household items, like rugs, pillows,
lights, and so on (see Figure 2.2). Extrinsic factors theoretically include everything in the household environment.

Data from the U.S. Consumer Product Safety Commission indicate that in 2010, 40 percent or more of emergency room treated
injuries that were associated with the products listed in Table 2.1
happened to people 65 or older. The data also show that falls were a
common injury pattern. The list is arranged in order of decreasing
number of injuries to people 65 or older. The number of injuries
associated with a certain category of product is then shown as a
percentage of all injuries associated with that product, regardless
of the person's age. An expanded list appears in Appendix A and
includes products for which 25 percent or more of emergency
room treated injuries associated with those products happened to
people 65 or older.

Other household items often associated with falls among older
persons include beds, bedding, clothing, and telephones. Some
other sources of fall risk are inappropriate footwear, low chairs,
dim lighting, bifocal or progressive eyeglass lenses, and pets.

The goal of this section is to help you identify relevant extrinsic
factors that could contribute to the risk of falls in your home. If
you prefer, you can obtain an evaluation specific to your home by
employing a professional home-hazard assessment service. A systematic way to identify extrinsic fall risk factors is to start physically
closest to the person (clothing) and move outward to furniture and
household items, going room by room. This is the pattern I have

used in organizing the following sections. (Chapter 8 contains illustrations of rooms and other areas that have been designed to
minimize the risk of injury.)

Table 2.1. Frequency of Product-Related Injury among People Ages 65 and
Older in 2010

Product	Number of injuries to those 65+	Percentage of injuries to those 65+
Crutches, canes, walkers	102,815	77% of 133,527 injuries
Wheelchairs	96,261	66% of 145,850 injuries
Toilets	54,080	52% of 103,998 injuries
Rugs or carpets	49,560	41% of 120,873 injuries
Runners, throw rugs, doormats	9,940	51% of 19,490 injuries
Recliner chairs	9,585	40% of 23,960 injuries
Step ladders	4,785	41% of 11,671 injuries
Electrical cords	4,030	40% of 10,083 injuries
Scales	1,306	55% of 2,375 injuries

Clothing

Thinking about tripping and falling hazards, focus on how you or
the person you are helping gets dressed and what the person wears.
Here is a variety of possible fall scenarios. These incidents each resulted in a visit to a hospital emergency room in 2010.

A 91-year-old fell backwards while trying to put on a pair of
pants.

A 75-year-old got a pants leg caught on a stair rail and fell down
the stairs.

An 86-year-old slipped and fell while wearing panty hose and
no shoes.

An 82-year-old tripped over untied shoelaces and fell.

A 65-year-old fell down two steps when the heel of her shoe got caught in a crack on a step.

An 83-year-old fell because of ill-fitting slippers.

A 69-year-old tripped on his robe while on the stairs and fell, hitting a radiator.

An 81-year-old tripped on pajama pants on his way back from the bathroom.

These incidents illustrate some important clothing-related issues:

- Getting dressed while standing may be dangerous for someone who has poor balance, especially putting on any kind of pants, which requires standing on one leg while engaging in a multipart activity.

- Belts or loose clothing can drag on the floor, get stepped on, or snag on hooks or other protrusions and create a tripping hazard or cause a person to lose her balance.

- Walking in just socks or stockings or wearing ill-fitting footwear can create a slip or trip hazard.

Here are two key questions to consider: Is the person able to get dressed alone safely or does he or she need assistance, and should the person get dressed from a seated rather than standing position? Strength, balance, and vision have to be very good for a person to get dressed in a standing position. If there are deficiencies in any of these areas, a chair is needed in the bedroom or dressing area. (Before making a decision on the kind of chair that will be most suitable, review the section later in this chapter on types of chairs.) Note that the suggestion is to use a chair, not the bed. As you will discover in the discussion on the bedroom, bed linens can make a bed a slippery surface; a bed can act like a slide for a person sitting on it.

Next, what clothing characteristics need to be considered? Figure 2.3 illustrates some common hazards.

HEMLINE

Take a look at pants, skirts, pajamas, nightgowns, and bathrobes, noting any part of the garment or related item (like a belt) that hangs near the floor. Make sure the garment always clears the floor when the person is walking. Clothing that drags along the floor can create a tripping hazard.

FITTED VERSUS FLOWING

Full, flowing clothing and dangling accessories can catch on other items and throw the person off balance. Look at sleeves, belts, belt loops, pant legs, and tops. Do they fit close to the body and not dangle?

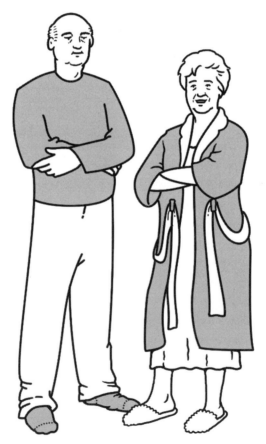

Figure 2.3. Clothing-related fall risk factors: pants that drag along the floor, stocking feet, dangling belt, and backless slippers

FOOTWEAR

Does the footwear provide support and fit well? Loose, ill-fitting, or very soft shoes, like slippers or moccasins, lack support and can create a tripping hazard. Shoes that are too tight or in any way make a foot hurt will affect a person's gait and balance. An older person should not wear shoes or slippers that are loose-fitting or backless. Daywear shoes should either lace up or close with Velcro® to be secure on the feet.

Are the shoes flat or do they have at most a small heel? Flatter shoes provide greater stability. Check the soles and heels. Are they worn out or in need of repair? Or should the shoes be replaced? Leather soles and worn soles can be slippery. Preferably, soles should be skid-resistant synthetic or rubber.

HOSIERY

Going barefoot or walking around in stocking feet is dangerous because there is less traction than when a person is wearing shoes. Feet must be comfortable inside shoes, and the kind of socks or stockings worn can contribute to comfort or discomfort. Hosiery that is too thin can make shoes fit too loosely. If hose have thinned from wear, parts of the shoe may rub directly against the foot, causing blisters, abrasions, or calluses. We have already noted that foot problems can affect gait.

NIGHTWEAR

Robes, pajamas, and nightgowns should not drag along the floor. Because a person might be shoeless at night time, or wearing slippers, the length of nightwear should be assessed on the assumption that the person may be shoeless. Make sure these garments clear the floor by at least 2 inches.

Climbing stairs can make clothing behave differently, so if there are stairs that the person must negotiate, take a look at how the clothing behaves on stairs. The hemline of nightgowns and bathrobes will probably need to be higher than you would think to account for people forgetting to lift the hem as they climb, *even if it's only one step.*

HIP PROTECTORS

While we are on the subject of clothes, I should mention that there is a garment that is specifically made to protect from injury during a fall. A hip protector is an undergarment worn so that in case of a fall the hip is less likely to be fractured. It works by absorbing or redistributing the impact of a fall. In one study, people who participated in a one-week trial of different brands of hip protectors reported that they found them uncomfortable, a poor fit, inconvenient, and unflattering. Few people in the trial spontaneously mentioned the protective benefits of hip protectors. A person's beliefs in the benefits of a hip protector will influence whether they choose to wear one. If a person is at a high risk for falling and has fragile bones, it would be appropriate to discuss hip protectors with her or his doctor.

The Bedroom

Since the bedroom is a typical place for people to get dressed, take a look around, keeping in mind the following reported incidents:

A 78-year-old who was getting out of bed got tangled in the sheets and fell.

A 73-year-old was sitting on the bed when the comforter slipped and she fell to the floor.

A 68-year-old tripped on a blanket, part of which was draped on the floor, and fell to her knees.

A 66-year-old who was changing the bed got caught in the sheets and fell.

To prevent falling out of bed, some people choose bed rails, but rails produce mixed results, and they can create hazards. A bed rail is an additional object into which an elderly person can fall while walking around in the bedroom. And they aren't always effective; some people actually fall out of bed over the top of the installed bed rail. Sometimes people become entrapped in the spaces of the bed rails (see Chapter 5, Figure 5.1). If the risk of falling out of bed is high, you might consider a hospital bed or similar bed whose height from the floor can be changed. Lowering the fall height might be the better solution, rather than installing bed rails.

As for the hazards associated with bedding, try to reduce the likelihood of entanglement by using the correct size linens for the bed. Use a fitted sheet for the bottom sheet and tuck in the top sheet, blankets, and covers so they do not dangle on the floor. When choosing the material for bedding, avoid satiny or silky textures, because these make the bed surface slippery. A person can slide off the bed onto the floor while trying to get into or out of bed, or while sitting on the bed trying to get dressed. (This is why a chair is a safer option.) Choose cotton, flannel, or blends that are less silky. Make the bed soon after you or the person you are caring for gets up; this will help keep the bedding in place, reducing the risk of entanglement and tripping.

The Bathroom

It doesn't take special training to see some of the fall risks in bathrooms. Toilets, showers, bathtubs, and scales all can pose risks. People lose their balance and fall when they are getting on or off the toilet. Grab bars or support bars can easily be added; they provide something to hold onto and help the person stay balanced while transitioning. A wide variety of designs is available. Raising the height of the toilet seat by using an accessory seat may also be helpful. These seats are sometimes equipped with handles, making it easier for the person to be guided on and off the seat.

Assess the ease of getting into the shower or tub. Grab bars will help, but if a person cannot easily step over the edge of a tub or shower, consider installing a walk-in shower or tub. These eliminate or greatly lower the edge the bather has to step over. To reduce the risk of falling once you are in the tub or shower, install grab bars and non-slip mats and consider using a shower seat. Shower stools or chairs are readily available, light weight, and easy to keep clean. Using a handheld shower head makes it easier for a seated person to bathe or be bathed; the water flow is easier to control for both seated and standing positions. Make sure that bathing needs—shampoo, soap, towels—are within easy reach. (See Figure 8.5.)

A scale can be a tripping hazard if it protrudes into a pathway, and getting on and off a scale requires good balance. If you have a scale, place it out of the walking pathway and position it near grab bars or some solid surface for the person to use as an assist to balance.

The bathroom will likely be used during the night by older people, so the path to the bathroom must be clear and sufficiently lit. You might have to think about rearranging bedroom furniture to make getting out of the bedroom and to a bathroom easier. Night lights can act as a guide in the dark, and a person can turn on additional lighting as necessary. Consider keeping a flashlight on a nightstand.

The Kitchen

Falls in the kitchen are often related to over-reaching. Reaching requires flexibility and precise motor coordination; reaching for far away objects can throw you off balance. To get at out-of-reach items, some people stand on a chair, some on a step stool or small ladder. Chairs can be unsteady and are not intended for standing. My mother once stood on a wheeled chair on a sloping tiled floor to reach an item in a kitchen cabinet! By some good fortune she was not hurt as the chair moved across the floor.

Older people should consider rearranging items in the kitchen cabinets so that those used often are well within reach. You might wish to buy a "reach stick," a special grabbing tool available at most hardware and medical supply stores. If you need to use a step stool, look for one with a handrail to help you keep your balance as you climb up and down. If you opt for a ladder, never stand on the top step. Invest in a sturdy step stool or ladder that is easy to open and lock in place. (See Chapter 8.)

Kitchen falls are also related to scatter rugs. It's best to forego them. Kitchen floors can be slippery, when wet with spilled food or drink, when being washed, or after being waxed. Clean up spills right away; let floors dry thoroughly after being washed before walking on them; and skip waxing.

Beware of kitchen and dining room chairs with loose cushions. Make sure the cushions are securely tied to the chair. Cushions may seem harmless, but when one 75-year-old woman sat down on a chair, the unsecured cushion moved and caused her to slip out of the chair and onto the floor. She broke her hip.

The Living Room

Rugs and chairs are the most common fall hazards in the living room. About half of all rug-related injuries occur among people 65 or older. The rugs that are problematic include runners, area rugs, doormats, throw rugs, scatter rugs, and so on, rather than wall-to-wall carpeting. The most common scenarios involve tripping and getting tangled in the rug, resulting in a fall to the floor. We can readily recognize why area rugs inherently present a trip and fall hazard. They can have fringe, cause changes in elevation of the walking surface, and they can gather and slide. The hazard can be exaggerated by a person's gait, type of shoe, degree of haste (as in hurrying to answer the phone), use of a walker or cane, and by the presence of extension cords.

Obviously, one can eliminate all hazards posed by rugs by removing all rugs. If this is not possible or desirable, consider each scatter rug, doormat, runner, area rug, and so on, then remove those that you believe pose the most severe hazard, whether because of their location (for example, in a frequently used pathway), condition (for example, frayed or unevenly worn), or design (having fringe or other decorative edging). For rugs you keep, add a slip-resistant pad underneath. If someone in the house uses a walker or cane or wheelchair, it is probably best to eliminate these kinds of floor coverings altogether. (See section on walking aids below.)

As for chairs, most reported incidents of falls involving them occurred when people were getting into or out of a chair or when a chair fell over backwards. Getting up or sitting down requires weight transfer, and weight transfer requires strength. To gauge the safety of chairs, look closely at the kind of chair, the area around the chair, and how the older person in question tends to sit.

- How high off the floor is the seat?

- Does the chair have arms?

- What material is the covering?

- Is the chair a recliner or does it have some mechanical features?

- Does the person use a pillow to sit on or at her back?

- Does the seat tilt backward? Forward?

- If the person falls getting out of the chair, what might he fall onto?

- Look around. Are there nearby glass topped tables, sharp corners on tables, fireplace edges or andirons?

Chairs should be easy to get into and out of. They should have arms to help with stability while sitting down and getting up from the chair. The chair itself should not move, like sliding on the floor. Recliners may be comfortable once you are settled in, but getting into and out of them poses some particular issues for older persons. Recliners tend to be big, deep, and to require considerable strength to move from one position to another. They can be difficult to get out of, and people have fallen while trying to get out of them.

In deciding which chair is best, look at the seat area. Does it tilt backwards, forwards, or is it level? If it tilts backwards, that would add to the difficulty of getting out of it. If the seat is low or very deep, that too would add to the difficulty of getting into or out of it. Can the person's feet make solid contact with the floor while he or she is getting up? Good contact with the floor will add to stability.

Getting up quickly from a chair to answer the telephone is a well-documented fall hazard. Place a phone near your favorite chair. If that is not possible, use an answering machine and set it to respond on the least number of rings. Then, listen to messages at your leisure, without rushing. If you have a cell phone, keep it with you.

The General Household Environment

Refer again to Figure 2.2 as a guide for assessing your household environment. Also see Chapter 8. Since many falls occur because of tripping, start by looking at your floor. We addressed the issue of rugs above. Extension cords are certainly convenient equipment and are necessary at times, but you should make every effort to minimize their use. If you do use them, run them on the floor along a wall, not under a rug or anywhere that they might get under foot. Electrical cords in the walking path are an invitation to tripping, as the injury data attest. Electrical cords under carpeting have the potential to be stepped on, be damaged, and overheat. These conditions can lead to a short in the wiring and subsequent fire.

Do you have a dog or cat? Pets are wonderful. They offer companionship and entertainment and keep you involved. But, they can be tripped over too! Each year between 2001 and 2006, an estimated 18,500 people 65 or older were treated in hospital emergency rooms for falls associated with a dog, and about 2,500 for falls associated with a cat. The highest rates of injury were among those 75 or older. The majority of these 21,000 falls occurred in and around the home. Women were more likely than men to fall, and fractures were a common result of these falls. I'm not suggesting you give up your pet, but be aware of where your pet is before you rise from a chair and as you walk around.

Is your home an obstacle course? How many things do you have to walk around to get from point A to point B? Coffee tables are notorious roadblocks. Falls onto coffee tables result in a range of injuries. Consider replacing glass tables with wood; consider a table with rounded rather than sharp corners; consider end tables instead of coffee tables.

Clutter can also be a pathway obstacle. Clutter is a known tripping hazard, especially if it is on stairs. Stairs and hallways should remain free of newspapers, magazines, mail, boxes, shoes, and so on.

Are there changes in elevation as you navigate the home—perhaps one step up or down to a kitchen or living room or raised thresholds in doorways? Consider marking these points of change with contrasting colored paint or tape so they stand out, especially if someone in the house has diminished vision or poor balance.

Are all areas well lit? Rooms should have good, even lighting, and so should hallways and stairs. Dim lighting is a factor in falls, especially for people who have vision problems. Light switches should be available at both ends of hallways and at the top and bottom of stairs. This last feature is so helpful it is worth the expense of an electrician to add switches.

Examine stairs for loose handrails, worn or loose carpet, and worn or uneven steps; determine if repairs are needed. High-traction tread surfaces, which allow the soles of shoes to grip well, are recommended on stairs. Examine outdoor stairs. Be sure they also are well lit and have handrails. Are the stair treads textured to help minimize the risk of slipping in inclement weather?

Keep in mind these common tripping hazards:

- extension cords

- obstacles or clutter in a pathway

- uneven surfaces

- poorly lit areas

Walking Aids

Ironically, devices intended to assist a person in walking—canes, walkers, and crutches—can pose fall hazards, as Table 2.1 and Appendix A testify. A 2009 study reported that the most frequent fall-related injury associated with walking aids was a fracture and that 60 percent of the incidents occurred at home. Although more than twice as many adults use canes as walkers, walkers were associated with the greater number of falls, seven times as many as with canes. The authors of the study explained that some of the differences between cane- and walker-related injuries were due to the fact that people who use walkers are weaker, frailer, and have poorer balance and greater mobility limitations than do people who use canes. They also suggested that people may have trouble using walkers effectively.

You may think that walkers are easy to use, but they are not. There's a right and wrong way to move with them on level ground, to turn around, and to position the walker in order to be able to sit down on or get up from a chair. Thresholds, ramps, and curbs require skill to manage. It takes some time to learn how to "operate" a walker. Imagine the challenge for older people. My father was in his nineties when he first used a walker. He was still very skilled cognitively. I overheard the instructions for use of the walker given to him by the visiting nurse. I thought it was a lot to digest at once, even though he was given the opportunity to practice. With certainty I can say that he did not use the walker according to instructions; rather, he adapted the technique in a manner that seemed intuitive to him. Fortunately he never fell, but I saw the walker as a mixed blessing.

The report authors concluded that more research was needed into how to design better walking aids. They also pointed out that more information was needed about the circumstances preceding falls associated with walking aids, both to better understand the contributing fall risk factors and to develop specific and effective fall prevention strategies. Their concern was well placed: knowing how a person falls will guide us to better prevention strategies.

If you are considering using a walking aid or have been told you need to, choose one that is right for you, as advised by your doctor or a physical therapist or other professional. Then learn how to use it correctly. Ask about the right way to do things, and *practice*. Visiting nurses and the staff at medical supply companies can help. And remember that when you use a walking aid, you need more space around you as you move about. That could mean that objects that were not in your way before might become obstacles now. A little revision to your household environment may be necessary.

Many extrinsic fall risk factors have been identified in this chapter. The following list is a quick review of key prevention steps for each area discussed.

- ✓ Do a wardrobe check, eliminating or altering clothes that create a tripping hazard and repairing or replacing unsafe footwear.

- ✓ Make up the bed right away after rising, tucking in sheets and blankets so nothing drags on the floor.

- ✓ Install grab bars in the bathroom to assist with stability and balance, especially at the toilet and in the shower or bathtub.

- ✓ Reorganize kitchen cabinets, storing frequently used items within easy reach. As needed, invest in a sturdy step stool and/or reaching tools.

✓ Eliminate scatter rugs.

✓ Route electrical cords along the wall, not under carpet.

✓ Keep stairways and hallways well lit and clutter-free. Hold onto the railing when using stairs. Arrange furniture so you don't have to negotiate an obstacle course.

✓ If you need a cane or walker, get instructions in how to use it correctly.

WHAT TO DO IF YOU FALL

In spite of all the prevention measures you take, you still could fall. If you fall and remain conscious, try to relax and take a reading of your body to decide if you can get up. Wiggle your fingers and toes, and take a few full and slow breaths. If you can call for help, do so. Don't rush to get up. Getting up quickly or the wrong way could make an injury worse. If you feel that you can get up by yourself, follow the directions given below and illustrated in Figure 2.4 to help you do that safely.

First, look around for a sturdy piece of furniture you can sit on or the bottom of a staircase. Don't try to stand up without support. We use a chair as an example in the illustrations.

1. Roll onto your side: turn your head in the direction you want to roll (towards the chair); roll over onto your side by moving first your shoulders, then arm, hips, and finally lift your leg over.

2. Use your upward arm and hand, followed by help from the lower arm and hand, to push up to a kneeling position.

3. Slowly crawl to the chair.

4. Place your hands on the chair and slide one foot forward so that it is flat on the floor. Keep the other knee on the floor.

5. Slowly rise and turn your body to sit on the chair.

6. Sit calmly for a few minutes before trying to do anything else.

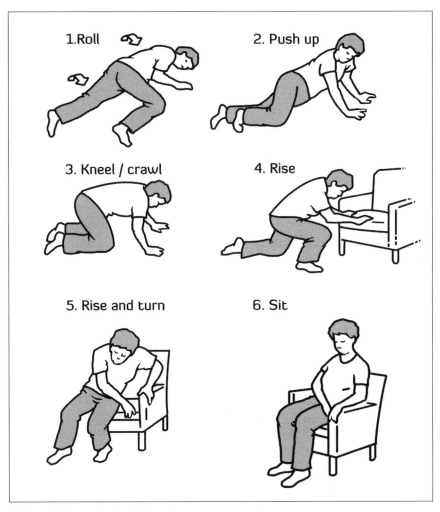

1.Roll

2. Push up

3. Kneel / crawl

4. Rise

5. Rise and turn

6. Sit

Figure 2.4. Getting up safely after a fall

Now, try to review, and if possible write down, what happened just before you fell and describe how you fell, so you can share this information with your doctor and others to help them understand why you fell. Note the date, time of day, and where you fell. What were you doing just before you fell? How did you fall—for example, did you trip over something or did you lose your balance? One study described four distinct kinds of falls: collapse (fall in a heap), fall in a direction (topple like a tree), trip or forward fall (failure to clear the surface—the foot catches on something), and sensory fall (insufficient sensory input for balance—for example, you took a step but didn't feel your foot touch the floor). Can you place your fall into one of these categories?

With this information, your doctor may be able to identify an underlying cause for the fall. Collapse can indicate a sudden acute condition, like a seizure, or a dramatic drop in blood pressure. This kind of fall would be a clue that intrinsic factors are involved. Falls in a direction are also likely to be related to intrinsic factors, for example an artificial hip slips out of its socket, or a person suffers a spontaneous fracture. A forward fall most likely reflects a trip over an obstacle and probably occurs while a person is walking. Tripping always involves an extrinsic factor, perhaps in addition to an intrinsic one. A forward fall may also be related to gait. A gait known as "freezing feet"—where the feet stop, but the body continues forward—forces a person out of balance, so they fall. A sensory fall is suspected when a person falls while walking (but does not trip) and experiences vertigo or dizziness. If an underlying cause can be identified, it will be much easier to correct the problem and avoid falling again.

You may want to consider a medical alert service to provide assistance in getting up after a fall. These types of services often incorporate a pendant- or bracelet-style help button that a person can press when he or she falls and cannot get up on their own. Some devices recognize when a person has fallen and automatically call for help even without the person's pressing the button. Some examples of medical alert services include: Philips Lifeline, LifeFone, and Medical Alert. An Internet search for "medical alert services" will yield several options to consider.

PERCEPTIONS ABOUT FALLING

A person's perceptions and beliefs about their risk of falling will influence their decision to undertake fall prevention measures and their commitment to following the steps they have chosen. Fall prevention should be encouraged as a way to promote health and maintain independence. If an older person believes that fall prevention measures matter, he or she is more likely to participate in prevention strategies and to do so with a positive attitude. If a person just expects to fall and doesn't think anything can be done to prevent falls, then that person will be less likely to accept that fall prevention measures will work, and thus will be less willing to participate in preventive measures. If a person thinks he or she isn't ever going to fall, it may be difficult to get that person to engage in fall risk assessment and undertake preventive measures.

Although falling can instill a fear of falling, it may still not motivate the person to take preventive steps. Family and community support for fall prevention helps older people recognize that falls don't have to be part of normal aging. Knowing that you have control over some fall risk factors will help reduce the fear of falling, as well. Fall prevention messages from public health organizations target seniors, urging them to focus on the positive health and social benefits of taking steps to prevent falls.

TO SUM IT ALL UP

Avoiding a first fall is the best way to minimize the risk of falls. Maintaining strength seems to be the major preventive measure one can take. It is strongly suggested that one incorporate several preventive measures, so you build a broad and diverse defense against falling. The following components are encouraged: exercises, particularly those for balance, strength, and gait training; modification of the home environment; minimization of medications; management of blood pressure and blood sugar; correction of vision and hearing losses; and management of foot problems and footwear. These interventions have been proven to be effective in decreasing falls and fall-related injuries. Adopting several of these intervention approaches offers the best promise of effective fall prevention. It is possible to prevent falls and, most importantly, injuries and death related to falls.

3

TOO HOT AND TOO COLD

Older people are at increased risk for burn-related injury and death. One reason is that our skin gets thinner as we age, and thinner skin provides less protection against burns and scalds. While superficial burns heal on their own, severe burns require medical treatment, can develop complications, and heal slowly. Older people also have reduced skin sensitivity and in addition, may not be able to move quickly, so they may not react to or be able to move away from heat or flame in time to minimize injury. The increased contact time with the burn source causes a more severe burn. Recovery may be prolonged and complicated by a change in living situation, if the person needs to be in a rehabilitation facility or any place other than at home.

Changes in the body and skin caused by normal aging also put older people at increased risk for hyperthermia and hypothermia. A reduction in the fat layer under the skin and the thinning of the skin mean that there is less natural insulation. If the body is not able to respond appropriately and adequately to external temperature conditions, extreme changes in internal body temperature can result. And they can be very dangerous. A dangerous rise in internal temperature is called hyperthermia; a dangerous drop in internal temperature is called hypothermia. Additional hyper- and hypothermia risk factors for older people include not realizing that they are too hot or too cold and being slow to respond appropriately to the body's temperature needs. For example, they may not promptly put on a sweater when cold or take a drink of cool water when hot. Older people may be less well nourished and thus have a lower metabolic rate; they may be more sedentary and thus generate less heat because they are not moving; they may be less well off financially and not able to pay for adequate heating or cooling.

Both ends of the thermal spectrum—too hot and too cold—can cause injury. This chapter is about how to prevent burns and how to prevent hypothermia and hyperthermia.

BURNS AND SCALDS

We can group the causes of burns into three categories: being burned through contact with open flame, being burned through contact with a hot surface, and being burned through contact with a hot liquid or steam. (Figure 3.1 shows examples.) Burns caused by contact with hot liquids or steam are called scalds. Contact burns and scalds may be minor (producing redness), moderate (blisters), or severe (deep, third degree), depending on how hot the surface or liquid you contact is and how long you stay in contact with that surface or liquid. The severity of open flame burns is related to how quickly and in what direction the clothing you are wearing burns, how long the flames continue to burn before being extinguished, how long it takes for emergency medical care to be administered, and how long it takes to reach a burn center for specialized treatment, if necessary.

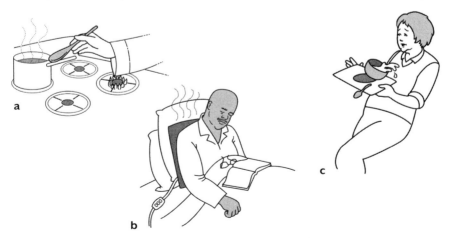

Figure 3.1. Three categories of burn: (a) open flame burn, (b) contact burn, and (c) scald

Burns caused by open flames are usually more dangerous than contact burns, because more surface area can potentially burn, as flames spread through clothing. Likewise, scalds are usually more dangerous than contact burns because more surface area can be affected and the contact period with the skin can be longer. If you touch a hot pan while taking it out of the oven, only the part of your hand in contact with the pan gets burned; if you knock over a pot of coffee, the hot liquid could spill down your pants and burn your legs; if you reach over a candle and your sleeve catches fire, the fire could quickly spread to encompass the whole torso. In addition, someone whose clothing is on fire may panic and run around, instead of doing the recommended "stop, drop, and roll." Someone who has spilled hot liquid on herself may not think to take the clothes off immediately or to pour cold water over the affected area. And, while it's usually easy to hold a mildly burned hand under cool tap water to prevent further injury, scalds and burns from open flames are not as easy to remedy and often require complicated treatment.

Burns and scalds most commonly occur in the kitchen, because that's where we cook, heat foods, and eat. But people also get burns and scalds in rooms with such products as space heaters, heating pads, hair dryers, irons, bathtubs, and cigarette lighters. A wide variety of circumstances can set the stage for a burn or scald. Here are some accounts of burns and scalds among people 65 and older treated in emergency departments in 2010:

Picked up a hot pot from the stove and burned hand

Reached over a stove to grab a pot and sleeve caught fire

Turned around while cooking at a gas stove and nightgown caught fire

Hair caught fire while blowing out a candle

Trying to light the furnace when a flashback burned the person's face

Backed into a heater and shirt caught fire

Fell asleep on a heating pad and back got burned

Burning trash in the back yard and pants caught on fire

Spilled boiling water, burning both thighs

Poured water on a grease fire, and the fire flashed up and burned the person's face

Frying potatoes while wearing oxygen equipment, and flames burned the person's face

How could these injuries have been prevented? That's the topic of the following sections, which are organized according to the three underlying hazards: open flames, hot surfaces, and hot liquids.

Open Flames

Factors that increase the risk of fire-related injury and mortality among older people include decreased mobility, hearing loss, loss of sense of smell, and confusion. Open flame is an obvious fire hazard. You won't always know that a surface you are near is hot enough to burn or that a liquid is hot enough to scald, but a person who is cognitively intact will always know that an open flame can burn them and can ignite nearby materials. So, the first exercise in creating a safer environment is to look for the use of open flame (including pilot lights) in the home. Some common sources are: gas appliances, including stoves, dryers, water heaters, and furnaces; lit candles; struck matches or lighters; fireplaces; grills; and woodstoves. We can add lit cigarettes, cigars, and pipes to this list, because they are often involved when bedding and furniture catch fire, leading to house fires.

THE KITCHEN STOVE

Open flame in the kitchen is likely to be limited to the oven and cook-top. The gas cook-top presents the highest risk of open flame hazard, and the greater danger is to the person who reaches near or over a lit burner. The best preventive measure one can take is to turn off burners before removing pans from them. The second-best preventive measure is to wear short sleeves, rolled-up sleeves, or tight-fitting long sleeves. Bathrobes, nightgowns, and tops with loose sleeves are an invitation to catching fire. Also, keep anything else that can catch fire—curtains, potholders, food packaging, towels—away from the stovetop. Note that electric stoves with coil-style elements can also ignite clothing and materials. Glass electric cook-tops do not present the same open flame hazard, although they do present the hazard of a hot surface.

The very first rule to do with kitchen safety is never leave cooking foods unattended! Unattended cooking is the leading cause of house fires. Stay in the kitchen while you are frying, grilling, or broiling food. If you are simmering, baking, roasting, or boiling food, check it regularly, stay home while the food is cooking, and use a timer to remind you that you are cooking, because it's easy to get distracted and forget about what's on the stove or in the oven. Many older people have a reduced sense of smell, which means they may not be aware that something is burning on the stove.

Hot grease can catch fire. If you expect there to be lots of splashing of hot grease, try to cook with a pot screen or pot cover and be sure to clean the stove after food preparation. Just in case, be prepared for a stovetop fire—keep a large pot lid nearby to smother flames. In case of fire, turn the stove off and slide the cover carefully over the flame. Leave the cover in place until it is completely cooled; resist the temptation to peek under it. *Never* pour water on a grease fire! It will *not* put out the fire; it will only cause the burning oil to splash, spreading the grease fire around. Never try to carry a burning pot outside—that will only slosh and splash the hot grease and increase burning and fire risks. A common recommendation is to keep a box of baking soda nearby and be ready to pour it onto a fire, but it may take a lot of baking soda to be effective. Covering the fire with a large lid is both quick and effective.

If you experience an oven fire, turn off the oven and keep the door closed. If that doesn't quickly control the fire, get out of the house, close the door behind you, and call 911.

OTHER GAS APPLIANCES

Many houses have a gas water heater and clothes dryer. Remember that these gas appliances have a pilot light—an open flame. If you store or use flammable liquids like gasoline, paint thinners, glues, and so on in the same area as the gas appliance, you are asking for trouble. Vapors from these products are highly volatile, and they are heavier than air, so they travel along the floor. Flammable *vapors*—not the liquid—are what first explode and catch fire. You won't see the vapors, but if they reach the pilot light, which may also be near the floor, they will ignite and explode. Store all flammable products in a different area from the gas appliance. Store gasoline in an out building or shed, not in the house or garage. All 30-, 40-, and 50-gallon gas storage-type water heaters manufactured after July 1, 2003 should comply with the American National Standard Institute's safety standard for water heaters and be equipped with technology to prevent the burning of these dangerous vapors, but it is still best to keep flammables away from flames!

If you have to relight a pilot light, be sure to follow the directions exactly. Not waiting a sufficient time between failed attempts to light the pilot can allow gas to build up. When you next strike a match, the vapors that have not had time to dissipate will ignite. This is how people get their eyebrows singed while performing this task. If that's all that gets burned, the person is fortunate.

OTHER PRODUCTS WITH OPEN FLAMES

Candles: Candles can be lovely and add warmth and pleasant scents to a room, but they also are an open flame hazard. Many candles have been recalled for posing a fire hazard because the candles themselves, not just their wicks, caught fire and set other items on fire. Some candle containers have shattered from the heat, posing not only a fire hazard but a laceration hazard. To completely remove risk from candles, do not have lit candles in the house; but if you wish to burn candles, do not leave the room they are in. Do not make a habit of keeping lit candles in several rooms at once.

I once was given a candle in the shape of a bird. When lit, the candle was supposed to shrink proportionally, keeping the shape of the bird. I lit the candle and set it down on a table that was covered with a tablecloth, intending to leave it there for only a few moments, then left the room. When I returned, the candle was completely on fire and so was the tablecloth beneath it! Had I gotten involved in, say, a telephone call while out of the room, my home might have burned to the ground. Lit candles should never be set directly on a flammable surface, and it's best to put the candle out when you leave the room and relight it when you return.

Fire pots: In 2011, fire pots that use gel fuel were identified by the U.S. Consumer Product Safety Commission as presenting an unreasonable risk of fire-related injury, because they can spread or spew ignited fuel onto users and surroundings. Unlike candles, these products do not have a wick to sustain the flame; the fire burns on the surface of the fuel. If these pots tip over while ignited, fuel and fire will spread very quickly. According to the commission, fire pots are

> portable, decorative lighting accents marketed for indoor and outdoor use. Their purpose is decorative. They provide some illumination and are not intended to provide heat. Many are made of ceramic material and look like vases or decorative pots, but some have different features and materials, such as a partial enclosure made of glass. Firepots are also sometimes called personal fireplaces, personal fire pits, firelights, or fire bowls. These products have the following characteristics in common. They: (1) are portable; (2) are open on at least one side; (3) have an open cup, usually made of stainless steel, to hold the gel fuel; and (4) are used with alcohol-based gel fuel.

Fire pots are relatively new products. They were not prominently marketed until late 2009.

The gel fuel used with the fire pots is viscous, like syrup, and is made primarily of alcohol so that it will burn clean, without smoke or ash. The most common injury scenario involving these products was a fire and explosion when the person was in the process of, or had just finished, refueling a pot that was still lit or warm. What happens is that the flame in the fire pot, which can be hard to see under certain circumstances, ignites the fuel vapor emanating from the spout of the gel fuel container as the person is pouring. The ignited vapor follows the trail of vapor back into the fuel container, causing an explosion inside the container. The explosion propels ignited gel fuel out of the container. Figure 3.2 illustrates this series of events. The ignited fuel can splatter onto people and things. Gel fires are difficult to put out with water, and patting the fire can spread the gel, which spreads the flames instead of putting them out. Two deaths and 86 injuries related to these devices had been reported as of December 2011. Several victims were hospitalized with second- and third-degree burns to the face, chest, hands, arms, or legs.

In September 2011, the CPSC recalled all gel fuels made by nine companies (Bird Brain Inc., Bond Manufacturing, Sunjel (2 Burn), Fuel Barons, Lamplight Farms, Luminosities (Windflame), Pacific Décor, Real Flame, and Smart Solar) and admonished consumers to stop using pourable gel fuel. As of 2012, the commission was considering what would constitute appropriate regulation of fire pots.

The fire pot refueling problems bring up a common pattern of flashback type burns: when liquid fuel is added to an already lit or still hot or warm fire (as in a fire pit, BBQ grill, or trash fire) the fire can ignite the vapor trail of the fuel back toward its container, and thus toward the person holding the container. Once a fire is going, even if it is not going well, do not add liquid fuel to it. Instead, add kindling or paper—that is, products that do not emit flammable or explosive vapors.

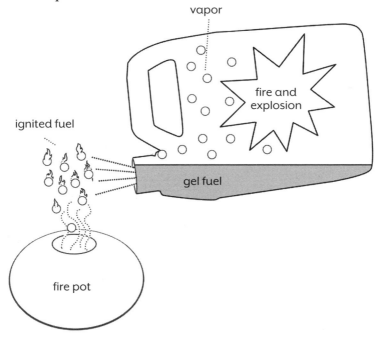

Figure 3.2. How fuel can ignite during refueling of a gel pot

Fireplaces and woodstoves: Also warming and lovely are fireplaces and woodstoves. Of course, we do leave rooms in which these types of fires are burning. In the case of these products, you want to make sure that the fire, including sparks and embers, stays inside, where it's supposed to be. This means having an adequate screen in front of a fireplace, and keeping the doors to the woodstove properly closed. You should also take some safety measures when trying to start a fireplace or woodstove fire. Use a commercially available fire starter log or newspaper and kindling to get a fire going, and gently add more wood over time to keep the fire burning. Do not over-load the fire with wood because the flame may get larger than you can contain. Do not use a flammable liquid to get the fire going. It has been reported that people have used gasoline or some other accelerant to get a fire going. This is extremely dangerous, as an explosion and generalized fire can occur. A fireball could envelop you. Never bring gasoline into the house; always keep it stored in a shed or out building. When it comes time to get rid of fireplace or woodstove ashes, make sure they are cool to the touch before discarding them in the trash. Many house fires have been started by warm ashes left in plastic bags or containers on decks, or near other flammable materials.

SMOKING

Smoking remains a substantial cause of house fires. Careless smok-ing accounts for one-third of fire-related deaths to persons over age 70. People fall asleep while smoking, causing bedding, chairs, or rugs to catch fire; people also empty ash trays while the ashes are still warm, causing trash containers to catch fire. If you must smoke, do not light up or smoke while in bed; and before you go to bed, thoroughly check for smoldering cigarette butts or ashes on any furniture you used during the evening—chairs, sofas, end ta-bles, coffee tables, etc. When you empty ashtrays, either dispose of the ashes into an empty metal can or let them cool overnight before you dispose of them.

There are many common products in the home that can ignite and should never be used while you are smoking or anywhere near an open flame. Know which household products are flammable. Some that we take for granted as safe and use liberally are quite flammable, for example, acetone-based nail polish remover, rubbing alcohol, certain hair sprays, petroleum-based lip balms and lotions, and certain glues. Read product labels carefully. Sometimes the information about flammability is in small, inconspicuous print. There is a federal requirement for flammable products to be labeled as such, so search the label thoroughly.

MEDICAL OXYGEN

There is another situation that becomes a very high risk for fire, and that is the use of medical oxygen in the home. The oxygen in tanks used for oxygen therapy is not like the air we breathe, which is about 20 percent oxygen. Medical oxygen is concentrated—it's 100 percent oxygen—and oxygen fuels fires. When the amount of oxygen in a room is increased, objects like furniture, clothes, bedding, plastic, and hair absorb the oxygen and therefore can catch fire at a lower temperature than they ordinarily would. Any fire that starts in the presence of extra oxygen will burn hotter and faster than usual. Even an oxygen tank that is turned off presents a risk.

Smoking while using oxygen is by far the leading culprit in house fires associated with oxygen use. These fires typically start in a bedroom or living room. There is no safe way to smoke if you use home oxygen. However, if you must smoke, there is a less dangerous way: shut off the oxygen, wait ten minutes, then go outside to smoke. This way, you will not continue to add oxygen to your clothes and hair, and when you go outside, the oxygen on you will dissipate more quickly into the larger atmosphere. When oxygen is in use at home, post signs inside and outside to remind others not to smoke.

Cooking at a gas stove while using oxygen and being around candles while using oxygen can also cause house fires, though cooking and candles were responsible for far fewer oxygen-related fires than smoking. Other products that can cause fires while oxygen is in use include, but are not limited to, electric razors (which can spark), space heaters, and hair dryers. Keep at least ten feet away from any flame or high-heat source while using oxygen.

OUTSIDE THE HOUSE

I love a steak on the grill. I am a charcoal person, myself, but any type of grill means fuel and fire. Familiarize yourself completely with how your grill works—how to light it and how to put it out. Follow the instructions every time, without short cuts. Never use fuel other than the one approved for use; never use starter fluid other than the one approved for use. You may be tired of hearing this, but based on the injury data I have reviewed, I cannot say it too many times—never, under any circumstances, use gasoline to get a fire going. After cooking is finished, if there are ashes to discard, wait until they are cool to the touch to do so.

Do you live in an area that allows backyard burning of trash or brush? If so, for the very same reasons mentioned above, do not be tempted to use gasoline to get the fire started. (For information on the hazards of burning poison ivy and oak see Chapter 7.)

In all cases, do not pour any liquid starter or accelerant onto a fire that is even warm. The vapor on the surface of the fluid can ignite, and the fire can travel up the trail of vapor to you.

What to Do in Case of Fire

If there is a fire, knowing what to do can make the difference between surviving and dying. According to the National Fire Protection Association (NFPA), from age 65 on, people are twice as likely to be killed or injured by fires compared to the population at large. According to the Consumer Product Safety Commission, those 85 or older are four times as likely. In an effort to reduce the number of fire-related deaths, the NFPA in conjunction with the U.S. Centers for Disease Control and Prevention (CDC) developed a program aimed at fire safety for older adults. They advise that, if you don't live in an apartment building, you consider sleeping in a room on the ground floor; this will make escape easier. Their program also includes these tips:

✓ Make sure that smoke alarms are installed in every sleeping room and outside of sleeping areas. The majority of fatal fires occur when people are sleeping; smoke can put you into a deeper sleep rather than waking you up. If anyone in

the house is deaf or has diminished hearing, consider installing a smoke alarm that uses flashing light or vibration to alert
to a fire.

✓ Have an escape plan and practice it (see second paragraph
below). Practice can help avoid confusion about what to do
in a fire.

✓ Make sure you can exit through doors and windows. Locks
should be easy to open. Windows should not be nailed or
painted shut.

✓ Keep a phone and emergency numbers near your bed.

Many households have smoke alarms that are not in working
order and thus will be totally useless if a fire breaks out. Make sure
all alarms have working batteries in them. The Consumer Product
Safety Commission recommends changing smoke alarm batteries
twice a year, when you change your clocks forward and back for
daylight saving time. If you are unsure whether or not you have the
correct number of alarms, ask your fire department to check your
home.

Having an escape route will help you get out quickly. Walk
through the house and make note of every possible exit and escape route. There should be at least two ways (counting doors and
windows) to get out of every room. Make sure the escape routes
are not blocked by furniture or other objects. Identify an outside
place to meet, a safe distance from the house, after the escape. Once
you're out, stay out! Under no circumstances should you ever go
back into a burning building. If someone is missing, inform the fire
department dispatcher when you call. Firefighters have the skills
and equipment to perform rescues. The NFPA website, nfpa.org,
has valuable fire safety information.

How to Prevent Electrical Fires

Some house fires are started by faulty electrical equipment or wiring. According to the Electrical Safety Foundation International,
electrical fires can be started by "arc faults." Arc faults occur when
electricity is unintentionally released from home wiring, cords, or

appliances because of damage or improper installation. This release of electricity can cause surrounding material to catch fire. The most common causes of arc faults are loose or improper electrical connections, such as household wiring to outlets or switches; frayed appliance or extension cords; pinched or pierced wire insulation, as could occur if a chair leg sits on top of an extension cord or if a pounded nail nips the wire insulation inside the wall; cracked wire insulation due to age, corrosion, or heat; wire insulation that has been chewed by rodents; overheated wires or cords; and damaged electrical appliances.

Have the home wiring checked every 10 years. Homes older than 40 years are more likely to catch fire electrically than those 11 to 20 years old, because old wiring may not have the capacity to safely handle new appliances and equipment. Technology continues to improve. Have an electrician examine your home. You may need more outlets, fuses, or circuit breakers; and unless you have circuit breakers from 2008 or later, you most likely need arc fault circuit interrupters (AFCIs). AFCIs replace standard circuit breakers in the electrical circuit panel. AFCIs can detect arc faults and shut down the power in milliseconds to prevent fires.

It's best to plug each appliance directly into a wall outlet and to avoid using extension cords. To reduce the risk of electric shock, have an electrician install GFCIs (ground-fault circuit interrupters) in places where water may be present. All bathroom, kitchen counter, outdoor, and garage outlets should be equipped with GFCIs. GFCIs monitor the amount of current flowing through an electrical outlet. If there is any imbalance, the GFCI trips the circuit, cutting off electricity and preventing shock and electrocution. A GFCI is able to sense a mismatch as small as 4 milliamps, and it can react in as quickly as one-thirtieth of a second.

You can check the GFCIs in your home to make sure they are working correctly by following these steps:

1. Press the "reset" button on the outlet.

2. Plug in an ordinary night light and turn it on. It should turn on.

3. Press the "test" button on the outlet. The night light should go out.

4. Press the "reset" button again, and the light should come on.

If the light failed to go off in step 3, have an electrician check out the wiring to the outlet, because the outlet could have been improperly wired or could be damaged, and if that is the case the GFCI will not offer shock protection.

Also, make sure that you use the correct wattage bulbs in lights. Lamps and other light fixtures are labeled to tell you the maximum wattage. Using higher wattage bulbs can lead to overheating and fires.

Hot Surfaces

Probably none of us has escaped the minor contact burn, the one resulting from touching a hot cookie sheet or a hot iron. Some of us probably have had more severe burns, say from contacting a hot engine muffler on a lawn mower. Very serious contact burns can result from contacting an extremely hot surface or from having prolonged contact with a hot surface, as in falling asleep on it or being trapped against it. Normally, our reflexes make us pull away from a hot surface quickly. Older people, especially those with diseases that affect peripheral nerves, like diabetes, may not have as keen a sense of touch and may not pull away as quickly. For them, contact time may be longer, and therefore the burn has the potential to be deeper and more severe.

Let's go back into the kitchen. Hot surfaces abound when we are cooking. Not only is the stove hot, but so are pots, dishes, handles, lids, and more. Check out the potholders. Are they in good shape, or worn? Do they offer adequate heat protection? Whatever the situation, adequate heat protection between you and the hot surface ought to solve the problem of contact burns.

Microwave ovens are a special case. Because the ovens themselves stay cooler than conventional ovens, we may not be on guard against burns when using them. Be aware that some dishes and mugs can become very hot in the microwave. Sometimes, the container gets hotter than the food. I have some microwave-safe dishes that behave exactly like that, so I no longer use them in the microwave. Always do a quick check for hot surfaces and use a potholder if necessary to remove items from the microwave. Stop using dish-ware that you know becomes excessively hot.

Place hot containers like pots out of your way and on a heat-safe surface, so you don't bump into them inadvertently while doing other tasks in the kitchen.

As for contact burn risks in other rooms, we have already talked about the open flame hazard of fireplaces and woodstoves, but these products also have very hot surfaces, as do gas fireplaces. The screens or glass doors on the fronts of these products can get very hot—as hot as 500°F. Keep your distance; if you have to move a screen or open a door to tend the fire, use a mitt or glove designed for the high temperatures these products generate. Because many young children have been burned by placing their hands on the glass of gas fireplaces, in 2011 concerned citizens filed a petition ask-ing the Consumer Product Safety Commission to require a warning on the glass and/or a safety screen.

Space heaters are sources of hot surfaces too. It might be tempt-ing, but do not get too close to space heaters; the heat they generate can ignite clothing. That's why they should be placed at least three feet from any material that could ignite, like draperies, rugs, and furniture. It's also a reason not to use them to dry clothes.

There are some additional concerns with fuel-burning space heaters (kerosene, gas, wood, coal) that do not apply to electrical heaters, because the fuel-burning ones generate carbon monoxide. If you must use such a heater indoors, take these precautions:

- Make sure the heater is installed by a professional, so that proper venting is achieved.

- Keep all the doors inside the house open, to provide good air flow.

- Turn the heater off when you go to bed.

- Install a carbon monoxide detector near where people sleep.

- Keep a fire extinguisher nearby.

Chapter 4 discusses carbon monoxide poisoning in greater detail.

Lastly, heating pads are worth noting as contact burn hazards. First-, second-, or third-degree burns can occur if someone falls asleep while using a heating pad, because one can be exposed to very high heat for an extended period. Sometimes heating pads are used in conjunction with taking a pain medication that causes drowsiness. This combination, and the fact that older people have a reduced ability to sense temperature change, can create a very dangerous situation. Keep heating pads at a moderate or low setting and use them for only short periods, not overnight.

Contact burn incidents associated with electric blankets are rare. Fires associated with electric blankets are also rare, but this tip should be followed: if you use an electric blanket, don't tuck it in around the mattress, for this can damage the wires inside it; and don't place additional bedding on top of it, because doing so can create excessive heat buildup, which can start a fire.

Hot Liquids

Scalds are particularly dangerous injuries, because typically more body surface is exposed to the excessive heat than in a contact burn situation. Also, trapped by clothing, the heat can stay close to the body for a longer time. Hot water has consistently been the most common source of scald burns—hot water from the tap, hot water from the stove or microwave, and hot drinks. Any liquid hotter than 120°F can scald; at 130°F, it will scald instantly. Since boiling water is 212°F, it's easy to understand why spilled pasta water, tea water, or any other boiling water is extremely dangerous.

Fortunately, scald injuries caused by hot tap water have diminished, because hot water heaters are now shipped from the factory with the thermostat set to a medium setting. Check your water heater thermostat; it should be set to a maximum of 120°F. Water heaters also are prominently labeled to warn about scald injury. Another protective factor is that mixing valves, which control the temperature of water as delivered at the tap, are more commonly used than in the past. Be in the habit of testing the temperature of water before stepping into a shower or tub. Because of reduced skin sensitivity, an older person using a hand to test the water temperature may not get an accurate reading. An easy way to be sure of the temperature is to buy and use a thermometer designed to test the bath water for babies. It will quickly register whether the water temperature is safe. This is very important, because if the water is too hot, impaired mobility and reduced sensitivity can mean that an older person is exposed for a much longer time to water that can scald and can therefore get a much deeper burn.

Spilled hot grease is a horrible scald hazard. The very high temperature of grease (350° to 400°F) can instantly cause terrible burns. Deep fryers present the increased risk of a larger volume of hot grease. If you use a deep fryer, be sure that the cord does not dangle over the edge of the counter. Inadvertent catching or pulling on the cord can pull the entire fryer, hot contents and all, off the counter and onto you.

Never store used grease while it is still hot; never pour hot grease into a container that can melt.

Hot wax from candles can also burn skin.

Fire and Burn Safety Checklist

Many heat-related hazards have been described in this chapter. They are presented in the following checklist of key prevention tips for minimizing the risk of injury associated with open flames, hot surfaces, and hot liquids.

PERSONAL

✓ Clothing: Wear tops with close-fitting sleeves or roll-up the sleeves.

✓ Bathing: Appropriate bathing temperature is around 100°F; test water before getting in, and set your water heater to a maximum of 120°F.

✓ Smoking: Never smoke in bed or around medical oxygen. Dispose of cigarette, pipe, and cigar ashes only when they are cold.

HOME ENVIRONMENT

✓ Candles: Stay in the same room with a lit candle; do not use flammables such as nail polish remover around candles; blow candles out when you leave the room or go to bed.

✓ Gel pots: Refuel with care and only when the product is completely cool; do not use brands of fuel that have been recalled.

✓ Fireplaces, woodstoves: Never use gasoline to start or fuel a fire. Be aware that surface temperatures of screens and glass doors can reach 500°F.

✓ Gas appliances: The pilot light is an open flame; do not store flammable liquids like paint thinners and gasoline in the same area.

✓ Electrical wiring: Have home wiring checked every ten years to be sure it is up to code and sufficient for your needs.

TASKS

✓ Cooking: Do not reach over open flames. Use good potholders. Be prepared for a stovetop fire by having a pot lid close by; never throw water on a hot grease fire. Keep stovetop clean of grease. Turn pot handles inward.

✓ Microwaving: Some containers will get hot; use potholders.

✓ Outdoor grilling: Use only the fuel recommended for the equipment; follow lighting instructions exactly. Dispose of ashes from charcoal grills only when they are cold.

✓ Backyard leaf or trash burning: Never use gasoline as a fuel to start or enhance a fire.

EMERGENCY PLANS

✓ Phone numbers: Keep emergency phone numbers handy and near the phone; program them into your phone.

✓ Exit strategy: Plan how to get out in case of a fire; practice the drill.

✓ Smoke and CO detectors: Install and keep in working order smoke and carbon monoxide detectors (in almost two-thirds of home fire deaths for 2005–2009, there was either no smoke alarm in the house or the smoke alarm was not working).

HYPERTHERMIA AND HYPOTHERMIA

Our bodies have their own thermoregulatory system. They are naturally designed to regulate our core temperature by keeping a balance between the heat we generate (when we burn calories) and the heat we lose (through our skin). When we are cold (losing too much heat), the body shivers to generate heat; when we are hot (not losing enough heat) the body perspires to get rid of excess heat. We also intentionally control body temperature by the clothing we wear, dressing more warmly in cold seasons and wearing lighter-weight clothing during warm seasons, and by adjusting the thermostat in our home for comfort. Average normal body temperature is 98.6°F.

Exposure for long periods to intense heat or cold can cause the body to lose its ability to respond to temperature change effectively. When the body temperature drops too far below (hypothermia) or goes too far above (hyperthermia) normal body temperature, we get into trouble. Both hypothermia and hyperthermia are dangerous. Hypothermia is defined as a body temperature below 96°F. There is no set temperature that defines hyperthermia, but concern grows as the body temperature rises above 98.6°F. A core body temperature of around 104° signals danger.

Older people are hospitalized and die from temperature-related illness at a higher rate than the general population. Some underlying health issues that can increase the risk in older people include poor circulation; inefficient sweat glands; skin changes related to aging; any illness that causes fever; heart, lung, and kidney diseases; high blood pressure; salt-restricted diets; inability to perspire related to taking certain medications like diuretics, sedatives, and heart and blood pressure medicines; being substantially overweight or underweight; and drinking alcoholic beverages.

Hyperthermia

The temperature outside or inside a building does not have to hit 100°F for you to be at risk for a heat-related illness. Heat exhaustion—a warning that the body is having difficulty keeping cool—and heat stroke—a medical emergency in which the body has dangerously exceeded healthy temperature—are the most common forms of hyperthermia. Here are some signs that mean a person may need relief. With heat exhaustion, the person may be thirsty, giddy, weak, uncoordinated, nauseated, and sweating profusely. The skin can be cold and clammy. If heat exhaustion is not treated, it can progress to heat stroke. Signs of heat stroke include confusion, combativeness, bizarre behavior, faintness, staggering, strong, rapid pulse, flushed skin, lack of sweating, delirium, and coma. Heat stroke is extremely dangerous and requires immediate medical attention.

Other heat-related symptoms include heat cramps, which involve a painful tightening of the muscles in your stomach area, arms, or legs. Heat cramps can occur after or during hard work or exercise. They are a signal that your body is getting too hot, even though your body temperature and pulse usually stay normal. The skin may feel moist and cool. Another symptom is heat edema, a swelling in the ankles and feet when you get hot. Finally, there is heat syncope, a sudden dizziness that may come on when you are active in the heat. If you take a medication known as a beta blocker or if you are not accustomed to hot weather, you are more likely to feel faint when in the heat. Pay attention to these symptoms.

Preventing heat-related illness is always better than treating it. Here are some steps you can take to help reduce the risk:

✓ Pay attention to the weather reports. You are more at risk as the temperature or humidity rises or when an air pollution alert is in effect.

✓ Dress for the weather. Natural fabrics (like cotton) tend to be cooler than synthetics (like polyester); lighter colors keep you cooler because they reflect the sun.

✓ During warmer months, especially if there is a heat wave, make sure there is enough air flow to keep the room temperature comfortable. Open windows can offer a cross-breeze, but if the only air coming in is very hot, you may need a fan or air conditioning (either central or window units) to help relieve the heat. At the beginning of the warm season, make sure these kinds of aids are available and working properly. If you do not have any of them, contact a local public health agency or council on aging to find out whether they have loaner programs.

✓ Keep shades and curtains drawn during the hottest parts of the day.

✓ If the home can't get cool enough to be comfortable, go someplace that is air conditioned.

✓ Drink plenty of liquids like water, fruit juices, and vegetable juices. Drink even if you are not thirsty. Avoid beverages containing caffeine and alcoholic drinks, because they help your body to lose fluids. If your doctor has told you to limit your fluid intake, ask what you should do when it is very hot. Avoid hot, heavy meals.

✓ Minimize or forego exercise or activities that can exert you when it is hot.

If someone is suffering a heat-related illness, here are some recommendations for what to do:

For heat exhaustion: Rest in a cool place, sponge off with cool water, and drink plenty of fluids. Get medical care if you don't feel better soon.

For heat stroke: Call 911. You need to get medical help right away.

For heat edema: Put your legs up. If that doesn't provide relief fairly quickly, check with your doctor.

For heat syncope: Put your legs up and rest in a cool place.

During colder months, make sure that the home is not kept at an unusually high temperature and that no one is overdressing so much that they could develop hyperthermia. While one is less likely to be on alert for hyperthermia in colder weather, lowered sensitivity to body temperature can cause older persons to keep the house too warm or put on too many layers of clothes and then not realize that they are too hot.

Hypothermia

Hypothermia is defined as a body temperature below 96°F. Hypothermia is dangerous because it can cause an irregular heartbeat, leading to heart failure and death. Signs of hypothermia include excessive shivering, confusion or sleepiness, slow or slurred speech, shallow breathing, weak pulse, low blood pressure, stiff arms or legs, poor control over body movements, and slow reactions. Because some of these symptoms can be related to other problems, just look for the "umbles"—stumbles, mumbles, fumbles, and grumbles—which show that the cold is affecting how well the person's muscles and nerves work. Observe the environment. Are you seeing these symptoms while the person is in a cold environment? Take the person's temperature. If it is below 95°, the situation is an emergency and the person needs medical attention.

If medical care is not immediately available, you can take these measures to begin warming the person:

- Get the person into a warm room or shelter.

- If the person is wearing any wet clothing, remove it and replace with dry clothing or covering.

- Warm the center of the body first—chest, neck, head, and groin—using an electric blanket, if available, set on low. Or use skin-to-skin contact under loose, dry layers of blankets, clothing, towels, or sheets. It seems a natural instinct, but don't rub the person's arms and legs—that can make things worse.

- Warm beverages can help increase the body temperature, but do not give alcoholic beverages. Do not try to give beverages to an unconscious person.

- After body temperature has increased, keep the person dry and wrapped in a warm blanket, including the head and neck.

- Get medical attention as soon as possible.

A person with severe hypothermia may be unconscious and may not seem to have a pulse or to be breathing. In this case, handle the victim gently, and get emergency assistance immediately. Even if the victim appears dead, CPR should be administered. CPR should continue while the victim is being warmed, until the victim responds or medical aid becomes available. In some cases, hypothermia victims who appear to be dead can be successfully resuscitated. If body temperature has not dropped below 90°F, chances for total recovery are good.

Preventing cold-related illness is always better than having to treat it. Here are some things you can do to help reduce the risk of hypothermia:

- ✓ Regulate the temperature of the home environment. How good is the home's insulation; is it intact? How old is the furnace? Is the furnace working properly? Does it need to be replaced? How well do the windows fit the window openings? Is too much air escaping or coming in? Do the windows need to be caulked or replaced? Are there storm windows? Is weather-stripping needed on doors? If heating the whole house is too expensive, could some rooms be closed off and not heated? The answers to these questions may not be obvious. You might benefit from a home energy evaluation, which can be performed by a local gas, oil, or electricity provider.

- ✓ Maintain good nutrition to keep the body's metabolism active. Balanced meals are key. How well-stocked are the fridge and pantry? Are there simple, easy-to-prepare meals at hand, like cans of soups, instant oatmeal or other hot cereal, and good-quality frozen dinners? Keep in mind that alcohol lowers the body's ability to retain heat.

✓ How about wardrobe: Are there enough cold weather clothes? Are there enough blankets and throws and are they within arm's reach of the furniture where they will be needed? Older persons should wear several layers of loose clothing. The layers will trap warm air between them.

✓ Manage diseases such as diabetes and thyroid dysfunction that affect blood flow or hormone levels. Are the medications being taken for such conditions doing their job? If not, they may need adjustment.

✓ Winter storms can knock out power, leaving the home too cold to be comfortable. Accessory heating systems, like space heaters may be necessary. If a generator is used, be sure to use it properly—it must be kept outside the house, to prevent carbon monoxide poisoning. Review the generator information in Chapter 4.

✓ Sometimes, a person's financial situation affects the risk for hypothermia. Most utility companies offer the option to spread out the cost of heating or cooling a home over the entire year; in some cases there is special relief for older people who need it.

Exposure to cold can also cause frostbite, an injury that involves freezing of the tissue. Sometimes frostbite and hypothermia coexist. The extremities—the fingers, toes, nose, and ears—get cold first, as the body channels its blood supply inward to protect the major organs from the cold. These are the body parts most susceptible to frostbite. Depending on the degree of cold, the length of exposure, and the layers of skin affected, injury can be permanent. The risk of frostbite is increased in people who have slowed blood circulation and among people who are not dressed properly for cold temperatures.

Any of the following signs may indicate frostbite: a white or grayish-yellow skin area, skin that feels unusually firm or waxy, or numbness. Because the frozen tissue becomes numb, a victim is often unaware of frostbite until someone else points it out. If you think a person has frostbite, get medical care for the person. As long as there is no sign of hypothermia, you can follow these steps until medical help arrives:

- Get the person into a warm room as soon as possible.

- Unless absolutely necessary, do not walk on frostbitten feet or toes—this increases the damage.

- Immerse the affected area in warm—*not hot*—water (the temperature should be comfortable when touched by unaffected parts of the body), or warm the affected area using body heat, for example, by placing frostbitten fingers in an armpit.

- *Do not rub* the frostbitten area with snow or massage it at all. This can cause more damage.

- Do not use a heating pad, heat lamp, or the heat of a stove, fireplace, or radiator for warming, because affected areas are numb and so can easily be burned.

Both hypothermia and hyperthermia are serious. If you are concerned about or responsible for an older person who may be at risk for being dangerously cold or hot, actually looking in on them will give you a more reliable assessment of their condition than a brief chat on the phone.

4

POISONING

Y ou would think that poisoning is a danger only for children, because most adults know better than to consume poisonous substances. But any substance can be poisonous if enough of it enters the body, and adults do get poisoned—as the public health data on poisoning attest.

The CDC (Centers for Disease Control and Prevention) defines a poison as any substance that is harmful to the body when ingested (eaten or drunk), inhaled, injected, or absorbed through the skin. Poisonous substances can include prescription and over-the-counter drugs, illegally used drugs, gases, chemicals, vitamins, and food. Poisoning is any harmful effect of being exposed to a poison.

The kind of damage caused by a poisoning depends on the poison, the amount taken, and the age and underlying health status of the victim. Some poisons are not very potent and cause problems only with prolonged exposure or repeated ingestion of large amounts. Other poisons are so potent that just a drop on the skin can cause severe damage. Some poisons cause symptoms within seconds, while others cause symptoms only after hours, days, or even weeks. Some poisons cause few obvious symptoms until they have damaged vital organs, such as the kidneys or liver, sometimes permanently.

Fortunately, most poisonings among older people cause only minor or moderate ill effects. A small percentage, however, cause serious injury or death. Of nearly two and a half million human exposures to poisons reported to sixty National Poison Centers during the year 2010, about 6.2 percent involved people aged 60 or older. About 0.2 percent of those older victims (232 people) died as a result of the exposure. But those 232 people made up 20 percent of all the reported poison-related deaths that year (232 of 1,146 deaths). Older people are indeed vulnerable to being poisoned.

Although children are more often poisoned by household products, cosmetics, and personal care items, older people are more likely to be poisoned by medications they are taking, whether they are prescription medications or over-the-counter medicines such as ibuprofen, acetaminophen, and aspirin.

What can we do to prevent poisoning of adults? The poison centers report noted that 93.7 percent of poisonings occurred at home, and we know that medications are the most common culprit of adult poisoning, so prevention begins at home with being careful about medications. Approximately 80 percent of the poisonings reported in 2010 were the result of ingesting a substance, rather than being exposed to it by other routes. Ninety percent of cases involved a single substance rather than multiple substances, and the most common substance reported was analgesics—pain killers.

This chapter focuses on medication poisoning, carbon monoxide poisoning, and food poisoning. Let me note right here that if you ever suspect a poisoning, you should immediately call 911 or the National Poison Control Hotline at 1-800-222-1222 for guidance.

MEDICINE: THE RIGHT DRUG, THE RIGHT DOSE

The term *medicine* includes doctor-prescribed preparations, be they pills, liquids, lotions, or whatever, that you have filled at a pharmacy; so-called over-the-counter, or OTC, therapeutic substances of any sort that you can buy without a prescription; and vitamins, herbal preparations, and dietary supplements. You should treat OTC medicines, vitamins, herbals, and dietary supplements the same way you treat medicines that require a prescription. Read the label, choose a substance that is appropriate for your symptoms, take the recommended dose, and follow the instructions for how to take the medicine. For example, if you have a runny nose but no cough, don't take a product that is for both cough *and* runny nose. Let your doctor know what OTC medicines you are taking, because they may interfere with prescription medicines you are taking. For example, if you take aspirin for a headache when you are already on a blood-thinning medicine, the blood thinner's effect will be amplified, because aspirin slows blood clotting. So, don't assume that just because a medication can be purchased without a prescription it can't be potentially harmful. This caution applies to herbal preparations, which many people assume can do no harm because they are "natural." In fact, they may require more care and knowledge on the part of the consumer, because they do not receive the same testing and regulation by the U.S. Food and Drug Administration that other drugs do.

Medicine-related poisonings are frequently caused by human error, such as taking a dose of a medication twice, taking the wrong medication, and taking the wrong dosage. Drug interactions are less common than taking the wrong medication or too much medication, but they are more likely than other medication mishaps to have a serious outcome. Drug interactions can result when the health professional makes a mistake in prescribing or when the patient takes more than one product containing the same ingredient. In the example of blood thinners and aspirin, the health care professional may not know when he or she prescribes a blood thinner that the patient sometimes takes aspirin, or a patient, having heard that aspirin can be helpful in preventing heart attacks, may add the aspirin on his or her own, not realizing it might cause problems with the blood thinner already being taken. Since many older people take several prescriptions (referred to as polypharmacy), they are more vulnerable to poisoning. (Chapter 2 explains the effects of polypharmacy on fall risk.)

Age-related changes in cognitive ability and loss of visual acuity can contribute to errors that lead to poisoning from medicines. If your memory is getting unreliable, you may forget to take a medication or forget that you have already taken a medication. If you have vision difficulties, you may misread a label and take the wrong medication or the wrong dose, mistake similar-looking containers or similar-colored substances and take either the wrong medication or a substance that isn't a medicine, mistake a hearing aid battery for a pill, or misread a measuring device and take too little or too much medicine.

Changes in fine motor skills can also factor in. People who have difficulty opening packaging (with child-resistant lids, for example) may transfer the contents to an unlabeled container to avoid the struggle. Transferring contents can easily lead to confusion about which medications are which. (And transferring medications or leaving off child-resistant closures can put at risk young children who live in the same household or who visit in the home.)

Recognizing the difficulty that older adults may have with child-resistant closures, the Consumer Product Safety Commission amended the Poison Prevention Packaging Act to maintain the same level of protection for children while at the same time ensuring that most older adults could open the packaging without undue difficulty. Child resistance is tested (by groups of children aged 42 to 51 months old) and now ease of adult opening is also tested (by groups of adults aged 50 to 70 years). A closure is considered child resistant if 85 percent of children tested *cannot* open it in a given time frame, and a child-resistant closure is considered effective for adults if at least 90 percent of older adults *can* open the package in a given time frame.

If you are confident that no children younger than 5 years old will be around, you can ask the pharmacy to fill prescriptions using non–child-resistant closures. These usually snap or twist on and off in one easy motion.

How Can You Help Prevent Medicine-Related Poisonings?

KEEP TRACK OF MEDICATIONS

Know what prescription and over-the-counter (OTC) medications you take or someone you are caring for is taking. Keep an up-to-date list of all prescription medications, including the dosage, the start date, the stop date, and the prescribing physician. Also keep an updated list of all the OTC medications and dietary supplements being taken, including the dosage, the start date, and the stop date. This information can help identify the problem drug if an overdose occurs. If you bring the list with you every time you visit the doctor, your risk of drug interactions or multiple prescriptions with the same ingredients is minimized. (See Chapter 9 for a sample medication record-keeping chart.)

Keep medicines in their original containers, so that you can identify not only the drug but also the pharmacy where it was obtained and the refill information. If you suspect a poisoning has occurred with that drug, the original packaging will be useful, because it has all the information you will need to report to emergency medical personnel or to a poison control center. If original contents are put into a different container, it's easy to forget what that substance is and what its medical purpose is.

STICK WITH ONE PHARMACY

If possible, use the same pharmacy for all your prescriptions. A pharmacy will keep a record of all your prescriptions and can alert you or your doctor to overlapping medications, contraindications, and potential adverse effects.

ESTABLISH A ROUTINE

Make it a rule always to keep the medicine in the same place (and out of reach of young children). Establishing a routine or habit helps you locate the medicine so you can take it on time. It also minimizes the risk of mistaking a different product for the medication.

It is very important to store medications in a separate place from hearing aid batteries and other small disc or coin-shaped batteries. Hearing aid batteries are exactly the same size as many pills. If a small battery is mistaken for a pill and swallowed, it can lodge in the esophagus or farther down in the gastrointestinal tract where it can cause chemical burns. Surgery might be required to remove the battery.

Take medicines at the same time or times each day. This helps regulate the amount of medicine in the bloodstream, for maximum effectiveness. It also reduces the chance of taking duplicate doses.

TAKE THE CORRECT DOSE

Make sure that you are taking the correct dose of each medication. Be sure to read the label. It will tell you how much to take at a time and how many times during the day you need to take the medicine. If you don't understand how to take the medicine, ask the pharmacist. The pharmacy's number is always printed on the label, and pharmacists are trained to answer patients' questions about medicines.

If pills have to be cut, use a pill cutter, which can be purchased inexpensively at any pharmacy. (An example is shown in Figure 4.1.) Cutting a pill in half without a pill cutter is not always easy. Some pills have a score mark on them (a line of slight indentation), which makes it easier to break the pill by pressing down on opposite sides of the line with your fingers, but other pills do not. Given the importance of accurate dosage and the potential for waste if a pill shatters while you are trying to divide it, a pill cutter is a very good investment.

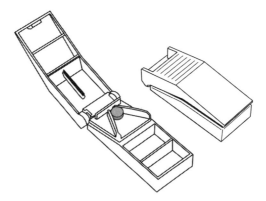

Figure 4.1. Pill cutter (a) open and (b) closed

For liquid medication, always use an accurate measuring device. An example of a so-called medicine dropper or medicine spoon is shown in Figure 4.2. These devices are marked with lines indicating the volume, and some have a mechanical device to make sure you pour to the correct line. Ordinary household spoons vary in size and should not be used as measuring devices for medicines.

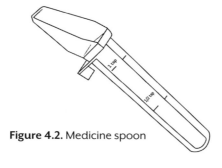

Figure 4.2. Medicine spoon

Using a pill planner or organizer can help you keep track of what you need to take when. Various designs are available, in different colors, with different numbers of days (see Figure 4.3 for an example).

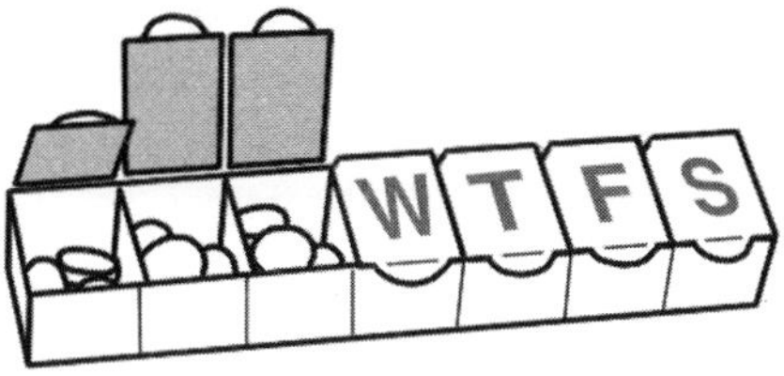

Figure 4.3. Pill organizer

Thoughtfully decide who will fill the pill planner. Correct filling of each slot is very important. Someone who understands the dosage requirements and can accurately fill the planner ought to do that task.

The planner should be refilled on a strict schedule. The day for refilling the compartments in the pill planner should be the same each week. There are at least two benefits to sticking to a fill schedule. First, a day's compartment is never empty when you need it. Second, when pills are running low, you have a trigger for requesting refills from the doctor or pharmacy.

Don't take a medication that was prescribed for another person. Even if the intent is well-meaning, doing this can create serious problems, including adverse reactions, overdosing, and allergic reactions.

In Case of Medication Poisoning

What should you do if you suspect a medication poisoning has occurred? The symptoms of medication poisoning are so varied, depending on the substance, that it may not be possible for a lay person to recognize them. Instead of waiting for signs of illness, if you suspect a poisoning call the National Poison Control Hotline at 1-800-222-1222 for guidance.

If you take someone to the emergency room with suspected poisoning, take with you the suspected substance or substances in their original containers. It would also be helpful to take the complete list of medications the person normally uses.

CARBON MONOXIDE POISONING

Carbon monoxide (CO) gas is poisonous. It is also colorless, non-irritating, and has no scent or taste. Those qualities make it an insidious killer—you cannot see it, you cannot smell it, and you don't realize it is causing you harm. One reason CO gas can quickly harm is that the red blood cells that carry oxygen throughout our bodies prefer carbon monoxide! That means, given the choice, they will select to absorb carbon monoxide over oxygen, depriving the body of the oxygen we need to survive. Thus, exposure to carbon monoxide is extremely dangerous and can be deadly. Symptoms of mild to moderate carbon monoxide poisoning may resemble flu symptoms. They include weakness, dizziness, nausea, and headaches. Symptoms of more prolonged exposure can include vomiting, loss of muscular control, and sleepiness. The most severe outcome of carbon monoxide poisoning is death.

Carbon monoxide is generated when any fuel burns, whether it's kerosene in a heater, oil or natural gas in a furnace, charcoal in a grill, wood in a fireplace, or gasoline in a car, lawn mower, or generator. That's why all fuel-burning devices are either designed and intended exclusively for outdoor use or, if intended for indoor use, are installed with a vent that leads outside the house. Electrically operated equipment does not generate carbon monoxide.

We cannot prevent the *formation* of carbon monoxide. The key to preventing CO *poisoning* is to make sure that the CO gets outside, into the air, where it can readily dissipate so that it is not available in concentrated amounts for anyone to breathe. With items ordinarily used outdoors, like lawn mowers, there is no real issue because as the CO is generated, it simply dissipates into the air. For items intended for interior use, like heaters, make sure that there is a vent to the outside and that the vent system is kept clean, clear, and in good repair. If the carbon monoxide can adequately vent to the outside, there is no cause for concern.

There *is* cause for concern when carbon monoxide accumulates, usually in a closed or confined space. If gasoline- or diesel-powered equipment is operated in a space that does not allow the CO to escape to the outside, there is always a risk of CO poisoning. Running a car in a garage is an example. Note that even keeping the garage door open will not safely disperse the carbon monoxide that is generated by fuel-operated equipment running inside a garage.

Carbon monoxide detectors have been developed to alert homeowners if carbon monoxide accumulates inside their home. As of November 2011, carbon monoxide detectors are required in certain residential buildings by 25 states (Alaska, Arkansas, California, Colorado, Connecticut, Florida, Georgia, Illinois, Maine, Maryland, Massachusetts, Michigan, Minnesota, Montana, New Hampshire, New Jersey, New York, North Carolina, Oregon, Rhode Island, Utah, Vermont, Washington, West Virginia, and Wisconsin). Many people do not know that their state has carbon monoxide detector laws, however, and many people do not install a CO detector because they don't know about the devices or don't understand how they work. Even if CO detectors are not required in your state, you should install one. They work just like smoke detectors except that, instead of detecting smoke, they alert you when there is too much carbon monoxide in the air. If you have questions, check with your local fire department.

About 20,000 nonfatal exposures to carbon monoxide occur each year in the United States. Carbon monoxide exposures are more likely to occur in winter months than in summer months, and most exposures occur at home. These facts are not surprising because the most common culprits are home heating systems, including furnaces, boilers, and other heaters. Winter storms pose a danger for stranded motorists who can be exposed to motor-vehicle exhaust, which contains carbon monoxide.

People who use portable generators at home when electricity goes out for any reason are also at risk. Because portable generators have been responsible for so many CO injuries and deaths, the U.S. Consumer Product Safety Commission requires that a carbon monoxide danger label (see Figure 4.4) appear on generators manufactured or imported after May 14, 2007. Never operate a generator indoors, in a garage, or in a basement. According to one study, more than half of people surveyed in 2005–2006 thought it was okay or weren't sure whether it was okay to operate a generator in a garage as long as a door was open, and about 40 percent thought it was okay or weren't sure if it was okay to operate a generator in a basement. *Always* locate the generator outside, far away from any vents, doors, or windows, so that CO gas does not enter the home.

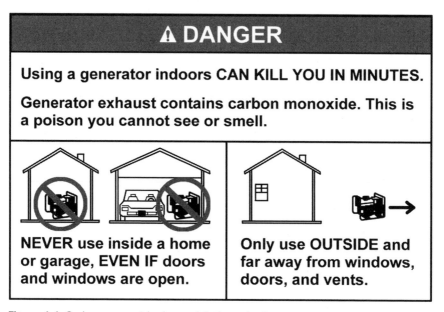

⚠ DANGER

Using a generator indoors CAN KILL YOU IN MINUTES.

Generator exhaust contains carbon monoxide. This is a poison you cannot see or smell.

NEVER use inside a home or garage, EVEN IF doors and windows are open.

Only use OUTSIDE and far away from windows, doors, and vents.

Figure 4.4. Carbon monoxide danger label required on generators

Adults aged 25 to 34 years had the highest rate of carbon monoxide–related visits to an emergency room, however, those aged 65 or older had higher death rates than the younger age groups. In 2009, 59 people 65 or older died from CO poisoning.

The consequences of carbon monoxide poisoning are also more severe for the older age group. Older people are more vulnerable because they are more likely to have chronic diseases, especially diseases that affect breathing. Also, the symptoms of carbon monoxide poisoning can be harder to recognize in older people because they may already have some of the symptoms of carbon monoxide poisoning, such as dizziness, for other reasons. In addition, older people might not be aware that their heating systems are operating incorrectly. If they are hearing impaired, they may not be able to hear the alarm of a carbon monoxide detector, or if they hear it, they may not know what it means or what to do, because of cognition problems.

How Can You Prevent Carbon Monoxide Poisoning?

Follow the precautions below to avoid this odorless threat:

- Make sure that any fuel-burning device used indoors is intended to be used indoors. Never burn charcoal indoors. Never operate a generator indoors.

- Make sure that any fuel-burning product used indoors, like a fireplace, space heater, or woodstove, has been installed by a skilled and certified contractor and is properly vented to the outside. Make sure that vents and flues are not blocked by animal nests, snow, or anything else.

- Have heating systems (furnaces) and fireplaces checked on a regular basis by skilled and certified contractors.

- Turn off space heaters when you go to bed.

- Never run fuel-operated equipment, including motor vehicles and generators, inside a garage. Even an open garage door will not allow the clearance of dangerous levels of carbon monoxide.

- Install carbon monoxide detectors in your home. Devices made especially for people who are hearing impaired emit visual cues or vibration in addition to sound.

What If You Suspect Carbon Monoxide Poisoning?

If the carbon monoxide detector goes off, open the windows and go outside. Then call the fire department for guidance.

If a person feels dizzy, nauseated, or headachy after using fuel-driven equipment in a confined space, lead the person outside for fresh air and call 911 for medical help.

FOOD POISONING

Each year, millions of people in the United States get sick from contaminated food. Some food is already contaminated when it is purchased, and some food spoils and becomes contaminated because it is too old or has not been properly stored. Symptoms of food poisoning include nausea, vomiting, diarrhea, and abdominal cramps. Symptoms can range from mild to severe and can start almost as soon as the meal is finished or as long as 72 hours later. For the most part, symptoms last a day or two and there is no long-term damage. In rare instances, food poisoning can be very serious and even result in death. If symptoms persist more than a few days or if the person has a fever or bloody stools, medical attention may be appropriate, especially to treat dehydration or infection. Harmful bacteria are the most common causes of food poisoning, but viruses, parasites, toxins, and other contaminants in food can also make people sick.

Age-related changes in cognitive ability and loss of visual acuity can contribute to errors that lead to food poisoning. Also, changes in the senses of smell and taste, a compromised immune system, malnutrition, and chronic diseases all increase the risk of food poisoning. Someone who is not able to see, smell, or taste accurately may not notice that mold has grown on an item in the fridge or realize that milk or another food has spoiled. (A person whose senses of smell and taste are poor is also at risk for malnutrition, because he or she can't taste the good flavor of the food and so may eat too little or have an unbalanced diet.)

Other contributors to food-related illness include improper cooking and storage of food and unsafe food handling behaviors, such as:

- Eating undercooked meat or eggs. Because eggs are relatively inexpensive, easy to fix, and generally well liked by older people, many older people eat eggs often, and sometimes they do not take care to cook eggs thoroughly.

- Not washing hands and food preparation surfaces thoroughly and often.

- Cross-contamination during food preparation, by failing to keep raw animal products separate from fresh produce. Cross-contamination happens when harmful microorganisms from uncooked foods (especially meat, poultry, and seafood) are transferred (by your hands, cutting boards, knives, and so on) to foods that are eaten without further cooking (like salad vegetables and fruits).

- Cross-contamination in the refrigerator due to poor or leaky packaging or storing raw animal products in close proximity to fresh produce. A leaky meat package may leak blood onto fresh produce or cheese, for example.

- Not washing fruit before eating it.

- Not refrigerating foods promptly when first purchased or when left over after meals.

- Thawing foods on the countertop instead of in the refrigerator.

- Keeping the refrigerator set to too warm a temperature.

A study of food safety practices done in England found that most participants had not measured their refrigerator temperature and did not know what the temperature should be. The study also found that the majority of the people had not adjusted the temperature control dial of the refrigerator and instead gauged the "correct" temperature by the feel of foods inside. "Use by" dates were generally well understood but not always adhered to because of difficulty in reading the labels. Items were sometimes purchased near the end of the "use by" date because they were cheaper and then, although people appreciated that these dates related to food safety, the items were kept for up to a month before they were consumed. If such a study were conducted in the United States, I venture to say that the results would be about the same. In fact, a Pennsylvania study of seniors who prepared more than five meals a week at home found that participants used a mix of inappropriate and appropriate practices in cooking, cooling, and thawing foods. Seniors relied on what they had learned in the past about food safety rather than on what is now known about safe food practices.

How Can You Help Prevent Food Poisonings?

Food safety involves a series of factors. Observing expiration dates stamped on packages is only one factor. The risk of food-borne illness is also affected by the temperature at which food is stored and the temperature of the room in which it is prepared. Focus your prevention efforts on these practices advocated by food safety experts:

Practice personal hygiene: wash hands and surfaces often.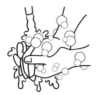

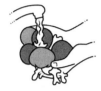 Wash produce before consuming it.

Shop where you trust the quality and safety of the food; be mindful of expiration dates.

Cook foods adequately: invest in a food thermometer and use it.

Avoid cross-contamination: in the refrigerator, keep foods separate and wipe up drips and spills so that foods do not contaminate each other. Thoroughly 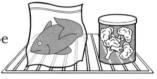 wash hands, food contact surfaces (such as cutting boards), sponges, dish towels, and utensils that come in contact with raw animal products.

Keep foods at safe temperatures and consume them promptly: Set the fridge to 40°F or colder. (If there is no digital temperature indicator, buy a refrigerator thermometer to check.) Quickly refrigerate perishables after purchasing, and store all leftovers in baggies or containers that close tightly or wrap them tightly in plastic wrap or aluminum foil. Use masking tape and a waterproof felt-tip pen to label containers and wrapped food, identifying the food and the date you put it in the refrigerator.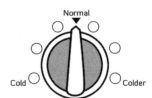

Foodsafety.gov is an online source of information on safe food preparation and handling. The recommended storage times from that website for various foods are listed in Tables 4.1 and 4.2. Note that food kept frozen remains safe indefinitely but that the *quality* of the food may decrease after the times noted. When freezing meat and poultry, wrap over the original package with foil or with plastic that is recommended for the freezer. Label and date items you freeze. Regularly review the contents of the fridge to discard items whose use-by date has expired. Thaw frozen items in the refrigerator, not on the counter, so that the temperature of the food does not rise to a level that invites bacterial growth.

Store canned foods in a cool, dry place. Never store canned goods under the sink, over the stove, in a damp basement or garage, or anywhere else that may have high and low temperature fluctuations. Canned foods with high acidic content, like tomatoes and other fruits, can be stored for up to 18 months. Low-acid foods, like vegetables and meats, can be kept for two to five years. Most canned goods now have "best by" dates stamped on the can.

Food safety experts offer this additional guidance:

- Generally, foods high in protein, like meat and fish, deteriorate faster than foods high in sugar or sodium. That's why sugar and salt are used in food preservation.

- Follow food safety temperature guidelines. At room temperature, bacteria grow quickly and food spoils faster. Refrigerate food soon after purchase. Keep your refrigerator set below 41°F and heat foods to temperatures above 140° F. These extremes of cold and heat prevent bacteria from multiplying.

- Take a good look! If you see obvious discoloration, such as green meat or blue spots on bread, throw out that food. Changes in texture are also a sign of spoilage, such as clumpy milk. Other warning signs are packaging with obvious openings or bulges, and cans that are dented, leaking, bulging, or showing rust along any seam.

How you handle food at the store, before it even reaches your kitchen, can affect your risk of food-borne illness. The U.S. Food and Drug Administration (FDA) recommends that, when shopping,

Table 4.1. Recommended Food Storage Times and Temperatures

Category	Food	In refrigerator (40°F or colder)	In freezer (0°F or colder)
Salads	Egg, chicken, ham, tuna, and macaroni	3 to 5 days	Do not freeze well
Hot dogs	Opened package	1 week	1 to 2 months
	Unopened package	2 weeks	1 to 2 months
Luncheon meats	Opened package or deli sliced	3 to 5 days	1 to 2 months
	Unopened package	2 weeks	1 to 2 months
Cured meat	Bacon	7 days	1 month
Sausage	Raw, made from chicken, pork, turkey, veal, or beef	1 to 2 days	1 to 2 months
Ground meats	Beef, turkey, pork, veal, lamb and mixtures of them	1 to 2 days	3 to 4 months
Steaks	Beef, pork, veal, or lamb	3 to 5 days	6 to 12 months
Chops	Beef, pork, veal, or lamb	3 to 5 days	4 to 6 months
Roasts	Beef, pork, veal, or lamb	3 to 5 days	4 to 12 months
Poultry	Raw whole chicken or turkey	1 to 2 days	1 year
	Raw pieces of chicken or turkey	1 to 2 days	9 months
Cooked meats	Cooked beef, pork, poultry, veal, or lamb	3 to 4 days	2 to 6 months
Soups and stews	With vegetable or meat added	3 to 4 days	2 to 3 months
Pizza	All kinds	3 to 4 days	1 to 2 months

Table 4.2. Recommended Storage Times for Eggs

Egg product	In refrigerator (40°F or colder)	In freezer (0°F or colder)
Raw eggs in shell	3 to 5 weeks	Do not freeze
Raw egg whites	2 to 4 days	12 months
Raw egg yolks	2 to 4 days	Do not freeze well
Hard-cooked eggs	1 week	Do not freeze
Casseroles with eggs	3 to 4 days	After baking, 2 to 3 months
Quiche	3 to 4 days	After baking, 1 to 2 months

you select refrigerated and frozen food after you pick up all the nonperishables on your list; that way, the foods that need to be kept cold are out of the refrigerated areas for a shorter time. (Most grocery stores are arranged so shoppers encounter nonperishables first.) Don't buy meats in torn or leaking packaging, and don't buy items beyond their "sell by" date or "use by" date.

To what temperature should food be cooked so that hazardous microbes are killed? It depends on the food, as the list below shows. If you don't own a food thermometer, buy one, because using a food thermometer is the only way for you to know the internal temperature of food. There are two types of food thermometers—those that you put into the food at the beginning of cooking and leave there throughout the cooking time (usually used with roasts) and those that you insert for a few seconds to get a temperature reading when you think the food might be fully cooked. The latter are called "instant read" thermometers; they show the temperature either on a dial or as a digital number.

The FDA recommends cooking foods until they reach the following temperatures, as measured by a food thermometer:

- Cook all beef, pork, lamb, and veal steaks, chops, and roasts to a minimum internal temperature of 145°F before removing meat from the heat source. For safety and quality, allow meat to rest for at least three minutes before carving or consuming. For reasons of personal preference, consumers may choose to cook meat to higher temperatures.

- Cook all ground beef, pork, lamb, and veal to a minimum internal temperature of 160°F.

- Cook poultry to a minimum internal temperature of 165°F.

- Cook fish to a minimum internal temperature of 145°F.

- Reheat leftovers to 165°F.

To see how well you are doing in the area of food safety in your kitchen, take the "Food Safety Interactive Kitchen Quiz" at http://homefoodsafety.org/quiz.

What If the Power Goes Out?

Food in the refrigerator will be safe during a power outage as long as power is out no more than two hours. During the outage, keep the fridge and freezer doors closed as much as possible. If the power is out longer than two hours, follow these guidelines:

- A freezer that is half full will hold food safely for up to 24 hours. A full freezer will hold food safely for 48 hours.

- For foods in the refrigerated section, pack milk, other dairy products, meat, fish, eggs, gravy, and spoilable leftovers into a cooler surrounded by ice. Inexpensive Styrofoam coolers are fine for this purpose.

- Use a food thermometer to check the temperature of food from the cooler right before you cook or eat it. Throw away any food that has a temperature higher than 40°F.

The rule of thumb for food safety is "when in doubt, throw it out."

5

PREVENTING ASPHYXIA

sphyxia is death caused by lack of oxygen. Drowning, choking, strangulation, and suffocation all can lead to asphyxia. In drowning, the person cannot get access to oxygen in the air because water enters the lungs instead of air. In choking, an object or food forms a blockage in the respiratory tract and prevents air from getting to the lungs. In strangulation, something wraps around the neck, making it impossible for air to pass from the nose and mouth into the lungs. In suffocation, something covers the nose and mouth or the position of the body interferes with breathing.

DROWNING

Of the four mechanisms, drowning is the most common cause of asphyxia among people 65 and older. In 2009, 545 people in that age group drowned. According to the death reports, about a third of them drowned at home, in either a bathtub or swimming pool; a much smaller number drowned in a hot tub or spa. In many instances, there was underlying heart disease, which means that the person may have suffered a heart attack and then drowned. In some cases, the person was not intentionally in the water, but fell in and drowned; for example, one man was skimming leaves from his pool and fell in. Some reports provided little detail on the circumstances, simply saying the person was found drowned.

The drowning prevention measures we take for children, such as fencing, alarms, and supervision, are not appropriate for adults unless the adults are cognitively impaired. However, a variation on supervision might be the best preventive measure for those 65 and older. This variation is the buddy system. An elderly person, especially if the person has a history of heart disease, should not be around a swimming pool alone. Drowning happens very quickly—usually within minutes—and very quietly. Contrary to what the movies show us, a drowning person does not splash or flail or call out. Therefore, waiting to hear sounds of distress or checking in on a person every so often is not nearly as effective as remaining with the person the entire time. Always have a working telephone by the pool, so that if an incident does occur, you can call for help right away. Take a first aid and an emergency resuscitation (CPR) course to prepare for drowning events. If there is a swimming pool on your property, such training is critically important.

There were a few drowning deaths in spas and hot tubs—about one for every five pool-related drowning deaths. Excess heat and alcohol consumption have historically been associated with spa and hot tub deaths—in all age groups. Always keep a thermometer in these products and check the water temperature before getting in. It should be less than 104°F. Immersion in water of a temperature above 104°F can lead to a variety of heat-related illnesses such as stroke, heart attack, nausea, and brain damage. Alcohol makes the problem worse. Thus, what starts out to be a relaxing scenario can turn fatal. A buddy system is recommended for spas and hot tubs, too.

Nearly half of the bathtub-related drowning reports mentioned underlying heart disease. Although no information on temperature of the bath water or length of bathing time was available, the hot tub and spa drowning information suggests that if bath water is too hot, it can be a complicating factor for drowning of someone who has heart disease. It is a good idea to check the temperature of bath water, too, especially if the bather has a history of heart disease or stroke. Bath water should be around 100°F, only slightly above normal body temperature. (Scald hazards associated with bathtubs are addressed in Chapter 3.)

CHOKING

Choking is a hazard primarily among the very young and the very old. Among older people, food is the common culprit. According to the National Safety Council, choking is the third leading cause of home injury death among those over the age of 76 and the second leading cause among those 89 or older. Not chewing food properly is the most common cause of choking. Older people may have reduced saliva and less than a full set of teeth, both of which affect chewing. Saliva and teeth are the essential gatekeepers—they prepare food for safe swallowing. Saliva moistens and softens food and eases swallowing. Teeth help control the amounts of food we bite off at once, and they prepare food to be swallowed by chewing and grinding it. Unless the food is properly chewed and ground, we may attempt to swallow a mass of food that is too big.

While dentures help make up for the loss of teeth, loose or poorly fitting dentures can contribute to choking. Although it happens rarely, dentures themselves can be choked on or swallowed. These factors highlight the importance of good dental care and evaluation as we age. (See Chapter 9.)

Meat products sit high on the list of problematic foods. Steak has a reputation for being difficult to chew, and was the most common restaurant food associated with sudden collapses of people while eating. These incidents, sometimes called café coronaries, were often erroneously thought to stem from heart disease; but the cause was choking, with meat blocking the airway at the back of the throat.

The same foods that are potentially hazardous for children because they lack a full set of teeth may be hazardous for older people: hard candy, peanuts, peanut butter, raw hard vegetables, popcorn, and hot dogs. Hard candy is slippery and hard to manage in the mouth; to avoid swallowing the candy as it melts requires sensitive control of the mouth, tongue, and swallowing reflex. Peanut halves and popcorn can be aspirated into the lungs, where they create chronic irritation. Peanut butter can be too thick to swallow without difficulty and can block the back of the throat. Hard vegetables cannot easily be chewed. Hot dogs, when not cut up into small cubes, are the perfect size and texture to block the airway.

Soft or pureed food and slightly thickened liquids are safer for people without teeth and people who have difficulty eating or swallowing. Other choking risk factors include eating too fast, drinking alcohol, taking sedatives, and having diseases like Parkinson's disease.

When planning menus for people at high risk of choking, avoid these foods:

- steak or big pieces of other kinds of meat

- hot dogs and sausages, unless you cut them into tiny cubes or lengthwise into thin strips

- popcorn, peanut butter, and hard candy

- very dry foods, like crackers and rice cakes

- large chunks of fruit, like apples or pineapples, or round slippery fruit like grapes

- thin liquids, like water (nursing homes add thickening agents to liquids to make them safer for residents who have trouble swallowing safely)

To help avoid choking, while eating we should all do the following:

- Do not talk with food in your mouth. (Talking requires air, so the airway is open. If you speak while you are chewing or trying to swallow, you could aspirate food into the airway.)

- Sit up; do not lie down or recline.

- Eat slowly, taking small amounts of food at a time.

- Chew each bite of food thoroughly before swallowing.

- Swallow food first, then drink.

Despite these precautions, choking can still happen. Look for these signs that a person may be choking:

- coughing or gagging

- clutching the throat or pointing to the throat

- sudden inability to talk

- wheezing

- passing out (loss of consciousness)

Everyone should know how to perform the Heimlich maneuver, though this life-saving technique must be done carefully in older people, who may be frail. The recommended procedure for the Heimlich maneuver—a way to clear a blocked airway—is as follows:

1. Call 911.

2. Get the person into a standing position. From behind, wrap your arms around the person's waist.

3. Make a fist with one hand and place the thumb side of the fist below the ribcage, just above the navel.

4. Grasp your fist with your other hand and press into the upper abdomen with a quick, upward thrust. Don't squeeze the ribcage with your arms. Confine the force of the thrust to your hands.

5. Repeat until the food is expelled.

If you are alone and choking, call 911. Even if you can't speak, call 911 and then leave the phone off the hook. In many areas, emergency personnel will respond to 911 calls when a caller doesn't speak. If you can, attempt to clear your airway yourself: thrust the middle of your abdomen (the area at the bottom of your ribs) against the back of a chair or railing.

Whether you are alone or someone else has intervened, seek medical attention even if you have cleared the airway, because the choking or the rescue maneuver could have caused internal damage.

SUFFOCATION AND STRANGULATION

Suffocation can happen in a number of ways: the nose and mouth may be covered, such as when the face is pressed against a pillow, preventing access to oxygen; the chest may be compressed, for example, if a person is entrapped between bed rails, preventing breathing; and in positional asphyxia the position of the body impedes breathing. One example of positional asphyxia is being seated upright but with the neck hyperflexed, usually forward, so that the trachea (windpipe) is compressed. Strangulation involves direct external pressure on the neck, usually by something wrapped around the neck, which prevents breathing.

Suffocation and strangulation are much less common than other types of injuries among older people. Only one strangulation death in an older person was reported to the Consumer Product Safety Commission in 2009. In that case, an 87-year-old woman's nightgown got caught in a nightstand. As she moved, the nightgown tangled and tightened at her neck.

Also in 2009, there were four suffocation deaths in older persons, three of which were related to entrapment in beds. They included entrapment between the mattress and a guard rail, entrapment within a guard rail, and entrapment in a bed frame. The fourth death resulted from entrapment between a bed and a nightstand. These patterns suggest that falling out of bed is an underlying factor, and that guard rails—while intended to prevent the person from falling out of bed—may introduce an entrapment hazard.

When guard rails are used on a bed, they must fit correctly and be designed for adult use. Installation instructions must be followed exactly so that no hazardous gaps are created. Figure 5.1 indicates seven potential entrapment areas on hospital beds, as identified by the U.S. Food and Drug Administration. Use this figure as a guide for identifying and avoiding hazardous gaps in beds and bed rails used at home.

Two compression asphyxia deaths were reported in 2009. One involved a dresser that tipped over onto a person, and the other occurred when a woman was trying to get into her home through a window and the window came down on her. (Compression asphyxia related to outdoor equipment roll-over is discussed in Chapter 7.) Two positional asphyxia deaths were reported. In one case a 100-year-old person collapsed on a chair, and in the other a 67-year-old fell off a chair and into a corner. Alcohol was reportedly involved in the latter death.

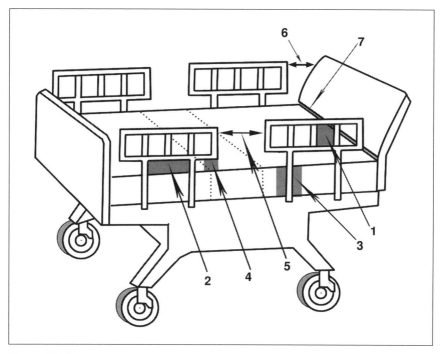

Figure 5.1. The seven entrapment danger zones in hospital beds as identified by the Food and Drug Administration:

1. within the rail
2. under the rail, between the rail supports, or next to a single rail support
3. between the rail and the mattress
4. under the rail, at an end of the rail
5. between split bed rails
6. between the end of the rail and the side edge of the head or foot board
7. between the head or foot board and the mattress end

6

WHEN DRIVING IS DANGEROUS

Driving a car means independence to most adult Americans; it means visiting friends and going to the store and seeing our doctors, without assistance and on our own schedule. By the time a person reaches age 65, he or she may well have been driving nearly fifty years. It's no wonder, then, that we take driving for granted! But the many changes that affect us as we age can make it unsafe to be behind the wheel. We may have to face the possibility of losing the freedom of driving. This loss is often frightening and nearly always frustrating. It may lead to isolation and depression.

Because people age differently, numerical age is not the factor that decides whether a person needs to stop driving; the person's driving capabilities do. All of the physical, sensory, and cognitive changes described in Chapter 1 can affect driving ability. If you search YouTube videos (youtube.com) for "older driver simulation," you can see interesting videos of how younger drivers, when physically adapted to be more like older drivers (by adding weights and restricting motion), find it very difficult to drive. These videos are eye openers, clearly demonstrating how the effects of aging can affect driving ability.

THE CHALLENGE FOR OLDER PEOPLE

Driving is one of the most complex, demanding tasks that we perform. In fact, it's the epitome of multitasking! To drive, we must process significant and varied sensory input, make countless decisions, and react appropriately, sometimes within a split-second time frame. We do this while simultaneously filtering out or dealing with distractions inside the vehicle and out. Given the complexity of the task, we should drive with all the focus and attention of an airline pilot or a cardiac surgeon! But we don't. Just look at the drivers around you. Not only are most of them engaged in conversation while they drive (the cell phone seems to be a permanent attachment to the ear), but they may be texting, reading a map, putting on make-up, shaving, eating, drinking, bouncing in their seats to loud music, and so on. No wonder motor vehicle crashes are the leading cause of unintentional injury death (when all ages are combined).

What effect do the changes that accompany aging have on driving ability? One example is that drivers with declining cognitive function and reduced control over attention may be particularly susceptible to distraction and therefore less safe to drive. They are more likely not to recognize landmarks and to get lost. Drivers with reduced sensitivity in their hands and feet may have difficulty steering or applying correct pressure to the accelerator or brake pedals. Drivers with visual perception deficits are more likely to be involved in rear-end collisions, because they cannot perceive depth accurately. Medications may make a person dizzy or sleepy at the wheel, and older people take more medicines, on average, than younger people do.

Injury data tell us that, mile for mile, older drivers are at similar risk for being in a car crash as are young drivers, however, when older drivers are involved in crashes, they are more likely than younger drivers to suffer more severe injuries, remain in the hospital longer, or die. The circumstances of the crashes older adults are involved in differ from those that younger drivers are involved in. Young drivers' crashes are more about risk-taking behaviors; older drivers' crashes are more about errors in perception or judgment. Young drivers' crashes often involve only their own vehicle; and speed, alcohol, or fatigue is likely to play a role in the crash. Older drivers' crashes are often multi-vehicular and happen at road junctions involving yielding to traffic, bikers or pedestrians, or changing lanes. In a comparison study of lane-changing behaviors between young and older drivers, older drivers were less likely to check the rearview mirror and blind spot before changing lanes. When forced to make lane-changing decisions quickly, older drivers did not increase the frequency of checking mirrors or blind spot, but younger drivers did. These types of omissions are cause for serious concern.

While sensory and cognitive decline are associated with aging, not all older drivers present a risk on the road. According to a 2008 article in the *Journal of Safety Research*, many people self-regulate their driving. That is, based on their own reduced confidence in their driving ability and on the fact that they enjoy driving less, they themselves reduce the amount of driving they do or alter the times of day and places they travel. The study reported that, when other driving options were readily available, such as another household member who could drive, it was easier for the older person to stick to his or her self-regulating decisions, because he or she could have the other person do all the driving or share in the driving. This way, the older person would not lose a sense of independence.

On the other hand, a 2011 study noted that, while self-assessments of driving ability may be used by drivers to decide how much they should restrict their driving, there remains a problem: many drivers have little insight into their own driving ability. Their self-restricting behaviors may, in the end, not be as beneficial to their road safety, and to that of others, as they think.

Ask yourself these probing questions to help you assess your own driving (or that of your parent, spouse, or friend who is an older driver):

- Do other drivers often honk at me?

- Have I had some accidents, even if they were only "fender benders"?

- Do I get lost, even on roads I know?

- Do cars or pedestrians seem to appear out of nowhere?

- Have family, friends, or my doctor said they are worried about my driving?

- Am I driving less these days because I am not as sure about my driving as I used to be?

- Do I have trouble staying in my lane?

- Do I have trouble moving my foot between the gas and the brake pedals, or do I confuse the two?

WHAT CAN BE DONE

Deciding when and how one's own driving or someone else's should be curtailed or stopped is a difficult and delicate process. Family discussions can be helpful if they focus on facts and aren't dominated by emotions. If family members begin to observe a decline in a person's driving skill, it is best that they openly discuss their concern with the person. Family members are often reluctant to try to convince older persons to modify their driving routines or to stop driving, because family interventions can become confrontational and lead to arguments, distrust, and feelings of being ganged up on. And they can have the opposite of the desired effect if the older person absolutely refuses to stop driving.

If family discussions are unsuccessful, and the family consensus is that the person is unsafe to drive—putting not only himself or herself at risk but others, too—consider engaging the person's physician in the discussion. The physician may be able to convince the person to stop driving; if a professional shares the responsibility for the decision, it can be easier for the older driver to accept. Moreover, physicians may need to report someone for unsafe driving to the registry of motor vehicles; some states require physicians to report medically at-risk drivers.

An objective, unbiased assessment of one's ability to continue to drive may provide the best help in the decision making. These types of evaluations provide outside-the-family help with one of life's toughest questions. Nobody wants to be the bad guy and have to tell a loved one to hand over the car keys once and for all. Fortunately, researchers have developed a series of tests that can be administered. Standard testing for driving ability considers vision changes, decision-making ability, attention, information processing, motor responses, muscle strength and coordination, range of motion, and medications being taken regularly. The tests are meant to be used as screening tools, not to determine, based on a score, whether the person should give up driving. Several tests are computer-based only; others have both a computerized portion and a road test portion. Some tests are conducted as an in-office doctor's visit. A few of the programs and testing options are described below.

The American Automobile Association (Triple A or AAA) and AARP (formerly the American Association of Retired Persons) provide online screening tools. AAA offers Roadwise Review, a free, online screening tool developed to help seniors measure certain mental and physical abilities important for safe driving. The screening tool takes about 30 minutes to complete, after which it helps identify and gives further guidance on the physical and mental skills that need improvement. AARP provides an online driver safety course for a fee. The program, which you can do at your own pace, includes: tuning up driving skills, updating knowledge of the rules of the road, and reviewing how to handle left turns, rights of way, highway driving, and blind spots.

The University of Michigan put out a driving decisions workbook in 2000 (available at http://deepblue.lib.umich.edu/handle /2027.42/1321). This is a 47-page booklet consisting of the following five sections, each of which deals with a factor that could affect driving ability: on the road (helps assess what factors add stress to driving); seeing; thinking (which includes hearing); getting around (personal mobility, strength, reach, and reaction time); and health (includes medications). Each section takes 5 to 10 minutes to complete and asks questions like "How much difficulty do you have following directions or a map in an unfamiliar area?" Based on responses, the booklet offers helpful suggestions, for example, "Plan your trip ahead of time and write down directions." Another example is, "Ask someone to ride with you to read a map or street signs."

Another program is DriveWise, a hospital-based driving assessment program developed in response to clinical concerns about the driving safety of individuals with medical conditions. This program, developed almost 20 years ago at Boston's Beth Israel Deaconess Medical Center and recognized as a national model, focuses on functional assessments to determine the driving competence of individuals of any age who have experienced neurological, psychological, and/or physical impairments. The interdisciplinary Drive-Wise team is made up of clinical social workers, neuropsychologists, and occupational therapists. They assess driving ability not solely on the basis of a medical diagnosis but on the individual's functional abilities. They might even utilize a certified driving instructor to conduct a road test with the individual; a skilled observer may ride in the back seat. If the program determines that it is not safe for the person to drive, the team takes steps to address the emotional needs of the individual whose driving safety has been called into question. In addition, the program helps identify alternative modes of transportation, so that the person's independence can be preserved as much as possible.

The ideal goal is to keep the person driving safely as long as possible, yet to take them off the road before they experience a crash. My father was involved in a car crash when he put his blinker on for a right turn as he approached a fork in the road. A driver coming out of a right-hand street before the fork assumed that my father would be turning onto that street, and so proceeded out of the side street, striking my father's car on the passenger side. Fortunately, no one was injured. After that, I used a subtle approach with my father. I frequently mentioned how expensive gas was, and he finally just told me to sell his car. I wasted no time and never asked if he was sure about his decision. I just moved forward very quickly with the sale of his vehicle. Of course, he had me to drive him places. Again, having another transportation option at hand can strongly influence whether the person cooperates.

No Longer Driving. Now What?

When a person, by choice or by persuasion, has to give up driving, there will be many consequences for that person and for those around him or her. The following questions will help you anticipate just some of those consequences.

- Who will be able to help with transportation? When and how often are they available?

- Will the person need to move to different housing to be closer to public transportation?

- Should the person move to an assisted living facility? Is that feasible financially?

- What will be the financial consequences of the person's not driving?

Talking with a social worker may help identify and solve the issues you are facing. Some areas offer free or low-cost bus or taxi service for older people. If you think taxis sound expensive, don't forget that it costs a lot to own a car. If you don't have to buy a car or pay for insurance, maintenance, gas, oil, or other car expenses, then you may be able to afford to take taxis or other public transportation. Some communities have carpools that you can join even though you don't have a car. Some religious and civic groups have volunteers who will drive you where you want to go. Your local area agency on aging can help you find services in your area. Call 800-677-1116, or go to eldercare.gov to find the nearest agency.

The Longer View

Because the number of older drivers will continue to rise, society must focus on the issue of making them safer drivers. The question will not be how to remove drivers from their cars, but rather how to keep older drivers mobile yet safe. Part of the answer may be in technology. For example: vision enhancement systems could assist visual impairment associated with night-time driving; improved mirrors could assist in eliminating blind spots; collision avoidance systems could help with speed and gap judgments at road junctions, avoiding backing up into objects or persons, and avoiding being too close to a curb; adaptive cruise control could help reduce the demands of challenging driving situations; redesigned foot pedals or the use of hand operated controls could help when foot sensitivity is compromised; adjustable foot pedals could enable very short people to drive while maintaining a safe distance from the steering wheel; and driver's seats that pivot outward would ease getting in and out of a vehicle. Some of these solutions are available now or will be soon.

While our goal is to keep older people driving safely longer, we need to realize that the longer people drive, the greater the chance they will be involved in a crash. One fact is certain: seat belt usage saves lives. Older drivers reportedly use seat belts more than any other age group. The most recent data available (2007–2008) show that about 85 percent of drivers 65 or older buckle up. Older adults with disabilities or in poorer health were less likely to use seat belts routinely. The reasons they gave included discomfort (feeling like the shoulder belt goes across the throat, or puts too much pressure on the chest); inconvenience; difficulty reaching for or connecting the belt because of pain, stiffness, or reduced flexibility; and obesity. Other factors include the type of trip (long versus short distance); road type (highway versus side road); vehicle type; who else is in the car; weather; concern that clothes will get wrinkled (especially fancy, dress-up wear, or material that wrinkles easily, like linen); resistance to seat belt use in general; and perceived low risk of a crash.

Some of the comfort issues have been addressed in newer vehicles by installation of a seat belt height adjuster on the pillar where the seat belt attaches to the car frame, but many older adults are unaware of this feature. Take a look there; you will easily recognize whether the seat belt height can be adjusted.

Another vehicle safety component that is not always positioned correctly is the headrest. The purpose of the headrest is to prevent hyperflexion of the neck in a crash. Unless the height of the headrest is appropriate for the person's seated head position, it will not function effectively. Go to the automobile's owner's manual. It will tell you how to adjust the headrest and what the correct position is.

Besides being involved in vehicular crashes, older people could be at risk for another highway hazard, getting lost. A 2010 study highlighted the seriousness of getting lost while driving. The study authors examined reports of drivers with dementia who became lost. Seventy drivers were never found, 32 drivers were found dead, and 116 drivers were found alive, although of those found alive, 35 were found injured. This highlights the importance of knowing when and where older drivers, especially those experiencing dementia, are going. Much as boaters or hikers leave their planned itineraries with officials, friends, or loved ones before heading out, older drivers should get into the habit of letting someone know where they are going and when they expect to return.

Automobiles are not the only transportation mode to be concerned about. A 2010 study noted that, among people 65 or older, motorcycle crashes increased 145 percent over the period 2000–2006. It is believed that the trend reflects, in part, a prolonged active life among the current generation of older Americans. According to Susan Baker, a coauthor of the study, "a 75-year-old person today is doing things his father probably would not have done at the same age." She also wrote, "Somebody once said that to move is to risk death, and not to move is to be dead already. I think there's some of that feeling among the current generation of older Americans." The elderly are also a growing proportion of all-terrain vehicle (ATV) operators. (Off-road vehicles are covered in Chapter 7.)

Safe Driving Suggestions from the National Institute on Aging

Here is some advice from experts on how to better manage the complicated action of driving a car while dealing with the added difficulties created by aging.

PHYSICAL CHANGES

As you age, your joints may get stiff and your muscles may weaken. This can make it harder to turn your head to look back, to turn the steering wheel quickly, or to brake safely.

What you can do:

- See your doctor if you think that pain or stiffness gets in the way of your driving.

- If possible, drive a car with automatic transmission, power steering, power brakes, and large mirrors.

SLOWER REACTION TIMES

In order to drive safely, you should be able to react quickly to other cars and people on the road. You need to be able to make decisions and to remember what to do. You may find that your reflexes are getting slower and that your attention span is shorter. Or, it might be harder for you to do two things at the same time.

What you can do:

- Leave more space between you and the car in front of you.

- Start braking early when you need to stop.

- Avoid high traffic areas when you can.

- If you must drive on a fast-moving highway, drive in the right-hand lane. Traffic moves more slowly there. Driving in this lane may give you more time to make safe driving decisions.

- Take a defensive driving course. AARP, American Automobile Association (AAA), and your car insurance company can help you find a class near you.

COGNITIVE PROBLEMS

Some health problems can make it harder for people of any age to drive safely, but there is no doubt that certain conditions more common among older adults make driving difficult. For example, Parkinson's disease, stroke, and arthritis can interfere with driving abilities. People with illnesses like Alzheimer's disease (AD) or other types of dementia may forget how to drive safely. They may also forget how to find a familiar place, like the grocery store or even home. In the early stages of AD, some people are able to keep driving safely, but, as memory and decision-making skills worsen, driving will eventually become impossible. If you have dementia, you might not be able to tell that you are having driving problems. Family and friends may give you feedback about your driving. Doctors can help you decide whether it's safe to keep driving.

What you can do:

- Tell a family member or your doctor if you become confused while driving.

- While you are still driving, always let someone know that you are going out in the car, where you are going, and when you expect to return.

- If you think you are still able to drive safely, contact one of the resources mentioned above that evaluates older drivers and sign up for an evaluation.

MEDICATION SIDE EFFECTS

Do you take any medicines that make you feel drowsy, lightheaded, or less alert than usual? Many medications can have side effects that affect driving ability. People tend to take more medicines as they age, so pay attention to how these drugs may affect your driving.
What you can do:

- Read medicine labels carefully (of over-the-counter as well as prescription medications), and pay attention to any warnings.

- Make a list of all your medicines, and talk to a doctor or pharmacist about how they may affect your driving.

- Don't drive if you feel lightheaded or drowsy.

SPECIFIC DRIVING CHALLENGES

Maybe you already know that driving at night, on the highway, or in bad weather is a problem for you. Older drivers can also have problems when yielding the right of way, turning (especially making left turns), changing lanes, passing, and using expressway ramps.
What you can do:

- When in doubt, don't go out. Bad weather like rain or snow makes it harder for anyone to drive. Try to wait until the weather is better; for necessary trips use buses, taxis, or other transportation services available in your community, or ask a younger friend, neighbor, or relative if they can take you somewhere or pick up something you need.

- Look for different routes that avoid places where driving can be a problem. Left turns can be quite dangerous, because you have to check so many things at the same time. You can plan your route so that you make only right turns.

- Get your driving skills checked at one of the driving programs or clinics that can test your driving and also make suggestions about improving your driving skills.

- Update your driving skills by taking a driving refresher course. Some car insurance companies may lower your bill when you pass this type of class.

DIMINISHED HEARING

The loss of hearing acuity that often happens with age makes it harder to notice car horns, emergency vehicle sirens, and even noises from your own car. The problems of not hearing these sounds in time are obvious, but there are more subtle sounds that drivers almost unconsciously rely on to help them drive safely, like the sound of a car passing your car or the sound of road bumps that warn that you are veering out of your lane and onto the shoulder.

What you can do:

- Get your hearing checked. The American Speech-Language-Hearing Association recommends a baseline audiogram at age 50, followed by an audiology checkup every 3 years after age 50.

- Get hearing aids if you need them, and don't forget to wear them when you drive.

- Try to keep the inside of the car as quiet as possible while driving. The radio can be pleasant to listen to, but it divides your attention and it masks the sounds from outside the car.

- Pay attention to the warning lights on the dashboard. They may let you know when something is wrong with your car.

Some Additional Safety Tips

PLAN BEFORE YOU LEAVE

- Plan to drive on streets you know.

- Try to limit your trips to places that are easy to get to and close to home.

- Take roads that will avoid risky spots like ramps and left turns.

- Add extra time for travel if driving conditions are bad.

- Don't drive when you are stressed or tired.

WHILE YOU ARE DRIVING

- Always wear your seat belt.

- Stay off the cell phone.

- Avoid distractions such as eating, listening to the radio, or having conversations.

- Make sure there is enough space behind your car. If someone follows you too closely, slow down and pull over if necessary to let that person pass you.

- Make sure there is enough space between you and the car in front of you; allow one car length for every ten miles per hour you are traveling.

- Use your window defrosters to keep both the front and back windows clear. If you don't know how to use them, consult the car's manual or ask someone who would know.

- Keep your headlights on at all times.

CAR SAFETY

- If you are buying a car, get one with air bags—the more, the better.

- Observe how well your windshield wiper blades work and replace them when they stop providing a clear windshield.

- Keep your headlights clean and aimed in the right direction.

- If you have leg problems, think about getting hand controls for both the gas pedal and the brake pedal.

- Don't be embarrassed to ask someone else to drive you somewhere if you are concerned about your own driving.

MORE RESOURCES

Making decisions about your driving skills is hard, but you need to find the safest option for you and those who share the road with you. Here are some helpful federal and non-federal resources. (Note that federal resources have ".gov" at the end of their Internet addresses.)

AAA Foundation for Traffic Safety
607 14th Street, NW Suite 201
Washington, DC 20005
202-638-5944
www.seniordrivers.org

AARP
601 E Street, NW
Washington, DC 20049
202-434-2277
888-687-2277 (toll free)
www.aarp.org

U.S. Administration on Aging
Washington, DC 20201
202-619-0724
www.aoa.gov

American Association of Motor Vehicle Administrators
4301 Wilson Boulevard, Suite 400
Arlington, VA 22203
703-522-4200
www.granddriver.info

Federal Highway Administration
Office of Safety—HSST
1200 New Jersey Avenue, SE
Washington, DC 20590
202-366-6836
http://safety.fhwa.dot.gov

The Hartford
Hartford Plaza
690 Asylum Avenue
Hartford, CT 06115
860-547-5000
www.thehartford.com
/alzheimers

7

THE BACKYARD
AND THE WORKSHOP

The backyard, the workshop, and the garage all are extensions of the home, and they harbor some of the same hazards that are found inside the home. They also present some special hazards.

YARD WORK EQUIPMENT

The backyard can be a peaceful place, with flower and vegetable gardens, trees and bushes, perhaps even a pool, pond, or stream. If you tend your own yard, chances are you water, mow, trim, plant, and so on. Gardening is a very popular and healthy pastime. Overall, it is a very safe hobby, too, but there are a few gardening hazards to avoid. In Chapter 2, I discuss fall hazards in detail. Although there are fewer risks for falling in the backyard than inside the house, they do exist. Here are some reported incidents:

An 89-year-old was raking leaves in his backyard when he tripped and fell, suffering a concussion.

A 71-year-old tripped over some rusty garden tools and lacerated his leg.

A 77-year-old fell when she pushed on a shovel as she was digging up a rose bush and fractured her arm.

A 75-year-old was weed-whacking and fell down an embankment.

A tripping hazard that sent about 4,000 people ages 65 and older to emergency rooms in 2010 was the common garden hose—a staple of gardens everywhere. What makes tripping on the hose potentially so dangerous is what the person might fall *onto*. The many possibilities include fences, raised garden beds, landscape timbers, railings, stone walls, curbs, and more. For example, an 83-year-old tripped over a hose in the garden and fell, striking his head on a brick, and a 93-year-old tripped on a hose and fell striking his head on a concrete flower box.

I am not going to suggest that you alter the terrain of your backyard, unless you feel it is particularly dangerous, but you can address the hose itself. Do you have it on a reel—so that it can be retracted and kept well out of the way? Help reduce the risk of tripping on the hose by rolling out only the length of hose you need and not much more and rewinding the hose after every use.

Mowing too is a reasonably safe endeavor, but we have all heard about people being injured from mowing. Mandatory federal regulations long ago addressed the once common hazard of a power mower's rotating blade lacerating or amputating fingers when people reached into the chute to clear accumulated grass clippings and inadvertently reached into the path of the blade. On today's power mowers, blades stop rotating when the user releases his grip on the handles of walk-behind mowers, or gets up off the seat of a ride-on mower. Many people understandably find these safety features irritating, but do not bypass them, because they really do substantially increase your safety.

There remains the hazard of tip-over, especially with ride-on mowers and lawn tractors. This hazard might not seem obvious. It can be hard to imagine such a heavy piece of machinery overturning. Tip-over can occur when the operator attempts to traverse land that is on an incline. The mower is thrown off its center of gravity and overturns. Tip-over can result in severe blunt trauma or compression asphyxia, as the rider usually gets trapped beneath the machine. In fact, 22 older people died in 2009 because of tractor tip-over. Review the user manual that comes with this equipment. The instructions will help you assess the incline of your yard and will tell you how to safely navigate the hills and valleys there. Correct technique is required even on the small inclines and dips.

Gravity is an ever-present force! Here's another example of how inclines can get the better of you: a 76-year-old was pushing a lawn mower down a hill when it gained speed, and as she chased it—or as it pulled her down the hill—she fell against a fence.

Running over bystanders, particularly young children, is another ride-on mower hazard. Children standing or playing in the yard while a ride-on mower is in use may not be visible to the operator, especially when they are behind him. It is such a tragedy to the family when a child dies this way. Never allow a child to be in the yard while the yard is being mowed; never invite a child to sit with you on a mower. These are not safe things to do. Even adult bystanders should stay several feet away from a mower to avoid being struck by thrown objects, like stones.

The hazards associated with gasoline storage and misuse are discussed in Chapter 3. Here I will talk about the hazard of gasoline while it is being *used,* not stored. Any gasoline-fueled equipment presents a risk of fire. If you spill gas while you are pouring it into the equipment's reservoir, wait a few minutes for the gas to evaporate before starting the engine, because a spark from the starter could ignite the gas vapors. When you need to refuel, wait a few minutes for the engine to cool, because spilling gas onto a hot engine could ignite gas vapors. And don't smoke or light up!

Ladders present the opportunity for injury outside as well as inside the house. If you are thinking of accessing those tree branches that need to be trimmed by using a ladder, you might want to reconsider and leave the job to a professional. Performing these kinds of tasks on a ladder is a good way to lose your balance. If you are using a power tool, like a small chain saw, instead of a manual tool, the risk for losing your balance increases. In addition, incorrect set-up of an extension ladder is very common. People tend to position the base (foot) of the ladder too far away from the vertical surface, which can result in the ladder "walking down the wall." On the other hand, if the foot of the ladder is too close to the vertical surface, leaning backwards while on the ladder can cause the ladder to fall away from the wall or tree or whatever it's leaning against, taking you with it. See Figure 7.1A for an illustration of the correct angle for setting up a ladder. Your ladder may have a label on the side showing an "L." This is to help you position the ladder correctly.

If you orient the ladder so that the horizontal leg of the "L" is parallel to the ground, it will be at the correct angle. If there is no "L" on the ladder, the rule to follow is this: Set up the ladder where you will be using it. Imagine a triangle drawn from the foot of the ladder to the point where the ladder is resting on something above and from that point straight down to the ground, then along the ground back to the ladder foot (see Figure 7.1A). That last line, back to the foot, should be one-fourth the length of the first line, from the foot up to the point of support at the top. You may wish to tape a copy of Figure 7.1A to the side of your ladder.

Another easier way to correctly set up an extension ladder is shown in Figure 7.1B. Rest the ladder against the vertical surface. Stand with your feet touching the base of the ladder and extend your arms. Adjust the ladder position until the palms of your hands rest on the ladder rung while your feet are touching the base.

Even correctly positioned ladders can topple if a person over-reaches. It is always safer to climb down and reposition the ladder than to reach too far to a side. One more thing before we leave ladders: if you are standing on a metal one or using a metal tool, be sure to be nowhere near a live electrical wire—look *up* as well as around before raising the ladder! Electrocution is a real and potentially fatal hazard.

Much of backyard power equipment is noisy—noisy enough to cause hearing damage. Wear ear protection. While we are speaking of protecting a sense, also think about your eyes. Wear eye protection to avoid being struck by thrown rocks or twigs while you are weed-whacking, mowing, leaf blowing, and generally using any power equipment to take care of the yard. If you chop wood, remember that striking tools, like mauls, axes, and so on, also can throw chips, off the tool itself or off the wood you are chopping. Wear eye protection for this task, too.

Do you want to power wash the deck or the siding? There are just a few things to be aware of. Most important is that water under that much pressure will cut through skin. Wear hard-toed shoes for this task; never wear sandals or shoes that leave your bare feet exposed. Follow the product directions to avoid an out-of-control wand. Once again, put on protective ear plugs and eyewear!

If you live in a place where snow is part of your landscape,

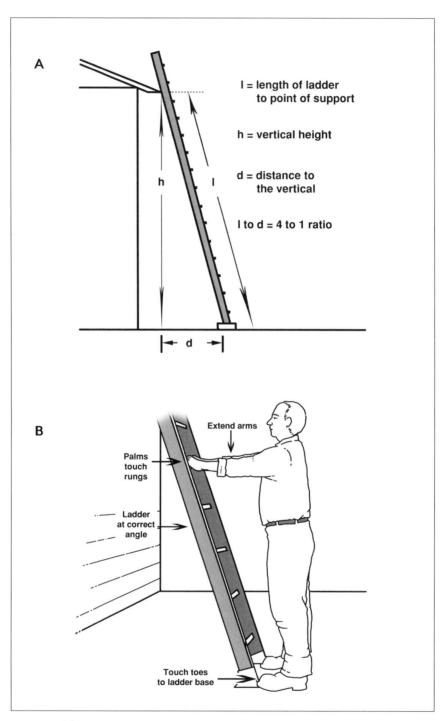

A

l = length of ladder
to point of support

h = vertical height

d = distance to
the vertical

l to d = 4 to 1 ratio

h   l

|← d →|

B

Extend arms

Palms
touch
rungs

Ladder
at correct
angle

Touch toes
to ladder base

Figure 7.1. (A) Mathematics of correct ladder set up and (B) easy method for correct ladder set up

perhaps you use a snow blower. In a recent study, older adults had a higher proportion of emergency room visits for injuries associated with snow blowers than younger people did. Most of the injuries to older people were finger or hand amputations associated with reaching into the discharge chute. The most common designs of snow blowers include a front auger that picks up snow and an internal impeller that discharges the snow from the chute. Both the auger and the impeller are rotating parts, and they rotate at high speed. Users who are not aware of the impeller blade and its location increase their risk of injury. If you use your hands to clear the discharge chute of wet snow you will be close to the impeller blades. Turn the equipment off and wait until the blades stop coasting before reaching into the chute. Better yet, use the cleaning tool that comes with snow blowers to clear the chute. It's a shovel-shaped device attached to the machine and is standard on newer models.

TROUBLESOME PLANTS AND BUGS

It's always good to know which plants might be poisonous. If you've ever had poison ivy, you know it is no fun. Poison ivy and poison oak are fairly common plants. Poison ivy exists everywhere in the continental United States except California; poison oak is primarily in the Southeast and on the West Coast. Poison sumac, another skin irritant, is found along the Mississippi River and boggy areas of the Southeast. Drawings of these plants are shown in Figure 7.2. As you look at the images of poison ivy and poison oak, remember this old saying, "Leaves of three, let it be." That guidance will help you identify these plants. As for poison sumac, look for stems that contain seven to thirteen leaves arranged in pairs growing directly opposite each other.

These poisonous plants are most often a problem when a person's skin contacts the sap oil that is released when the leaf or other plant parts, including roots, are bruised, damaged, or burned. The result is an itchy red rash with bumps or blisters. Most people will develop a rash after exposure to an amount of sap oil the size of a grain of salt. Depending upon where on the body exposure occurs and how broadly it is spread, the rash may need medical attention.

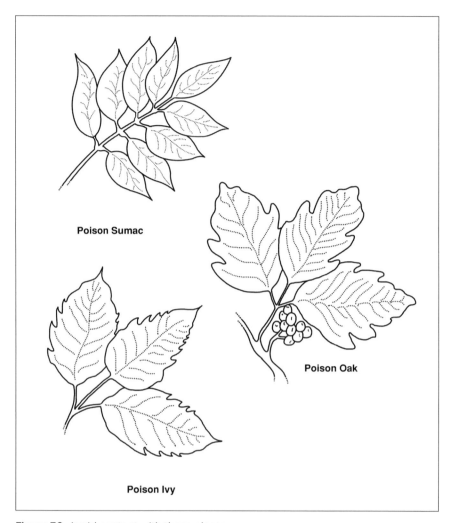

Figure 7.2. Avoid contact with these plants.

If you have been exposed to smoke from burning these plants, you should seek immediate medical attention, because the inhaled allergens will cause throat and lung irritation. For most minor skin exposures, an over-the-counter topical medication like calamine lotion or hydrocortisone cream may suffice. An antihistamine like Benadryl will help relieve the itching.

If you know you have any of these poison plants in your yard, avoid contact by wearing long sleeves, long pants, and gloves when working around them. When you are finished, wash those clothes separately—not with other clothing—in hot water, and any tools you used directly with the plants should be washed with rubbing alcohol or soap and lots of water. Wash your hands with dishwashing soap, because it is a degreaser, and you want to get rid of any sap oil on your skin.

Although ticks are more likely to be found in the woods or high grass than in your backyard, they are worth mentioning because of the potential for contracting Lyme disease. Lyme disease gets its name from the town of Old Lyme, Connecticut, where the first case was identified in the United States in 1975. Lyme disease is the most commonly reported tick-borne disease in the United States. It is passed to humans by the bite of black-legged ticks, also known as deer ticks in the eastern United States, and western black-legged ticks that are infected with the bacterium *Borrelia burgdorferi*. Deer ticks prefer to feed on the blood of white-tailed deer, but humans who brush up against leaves or grass where there are ticks can become unknowing hosts.

Black-legged ticks can be so small that they are almost impossible to see; many people with Lyme disease never even saw a tick on their body. So, if you are in a woodsy area or anywhere that attracts wildlife, especially deer, wear light-colored long pants, a long-sleeved shirt, and socks. This will help protect you and make ticks easier to spot. By comparison with black-legged ticks, wood ticks—which do *not* transmit Lyme disease—are much larger (see Figure 7.3). Wood ticks typically feed on the blood of dogs and cats, but they, too, will attach to a human. They are readily visible, however, especially if engorged with blood, and are thus more easily noticed and removed.

Not all black-legged ticks are infected with the bacterium and most people who are bitten by a tick do not get Lyme disease. The Lyme disease bacterium normally lives in mice, squirrels, and other small mammals. When a tick bites an infected animal, the tick can become infected with the bacterium. When that infected tick then bites a person, the bacterium can infect that person. In 2010, more than 22,500 confirmed and 7,500 probable cases of Lyme disease were reported to the Centers for Disease Control and Prevention. These statistics include persons who were exposed in the course of their jobs. The highest numbers of confirmed Lyme disease cases were reported from Maine, New Hampshire, Massachusetts,

Connecticut, New York, New Jersey, Pennsylvania, Maryland, Delaware, Virginia, Wisconsin, and Minnesota. If diagnosed and *treated early* with antibiotics, Lyme disease is almost always readily cured.

There are three stages of Lyme disease. Stage 1 is called early localized Lyme disease. The infection is not yet widespread in the body. There may be a "bull's eye" rash, a flat or slightly raised red spot at the site of the tick bite. Often there is a clear area in the center. It can be quite large and expanding in size. Symptoms can include body-wide itching, chills, fever, a general ill feeling, headache, light-headedness or fainting, muscle pain, or stiff neck.

Stage 2 is called early disseminated Lyme disease. The bacteria have begun to spread throughout the body. Stage 3 is called late disseminated Lyme disease. The bacteria have spread throughout the body. In most cases, a tick must be attached to your body for 24 to 36 hours to spread the bacteria to your blood.

If Lyme disease is not promptly treated, it can spread to the brain, heart, and joints. If you think you may have been moving around in areas where ticks abound, after you get home, remove your clothes and thoroughly inspect all skin surface areas, including between your fingers and toes and your scalp. Shower soon after coming indoors, to wash off any unseen ticks. Always check

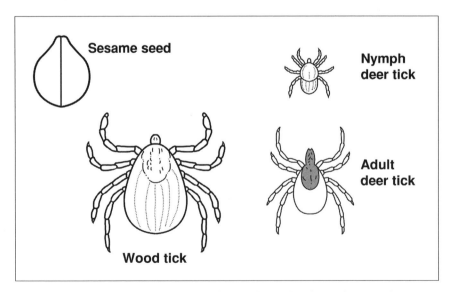

Figure 7.3. Comparative sizes of wood ticks and deer ticks; deer ticks spread Lyme disease

your pets for ticks, too. According to the American Lyme Disease Foundation, if you discover a deer tick attached to your skin but it has not yet become engorged, it has probably not been there long enough to transmit disease. Just in case, however, be alert for any symptoms (a red rash, especially surrounding the tick bite, flu-like symptoms, or joint pains) in the first month following any deer tick bite. If a rash or other early symptoms develop, see a physician immediately.

The American Lyme Disease Foundation recommends following these steps to remove a tick (http://www.aldf.com/lyme.shtml #removal):

1. Using a pair of fine-pointed, precision tweezers (with smooth, not rasped tips), grasp the tick by the head or mouthparts right where they enter the skin. DO NOT grasp the tick by the body.

2. Without jerking, pull firmly and steadily directly outward. DO NOT twist the tick out or apply petroleum jelly, a hot match, alcohol, or any other irritant to the tick in an attempt to get it to back out.

3. Place the tick in a vial or small jar of alcohol to kill it.

4. Clean the bite wound with disinfectant, such as alcohol or peroxide.

HOBBIES

Another extension of the home environment is the workshop or garage. If your hobby involves woodworking, you already know that woodworking tools have inherent hazards, like fast moving blades, sharp edges, and sharp points—all of which are necessary for the tool to do its job well. Two common blade-related injuries often associated with table saws, circular saws, and radial arm saws, are kickback and inadvertent contact with the blade. Both can result in very severe injury or even death. Kickback can cause internal injuries, as well as external lacerations. Correct feeding of materials into the blade and correct body positioning can reduce the risk of kickback type injuries. The use of guards on the saw can reduce the risk of inadvertent contact with the blade. And, of course, you will be wearing protection for your eyes and ears.

In 2010, about 10,000 people older than 65 were treated in hospital emergency departments for injuries sustained while operating table or bench saws. Most of the injuries were hand or finger lacerations or amputations. If your equipment has a guard (and it should), I encourage you to use the guard in its proper position. The Consumer Product Safety Commission is considering (in 2013) whether a new mandatory performance safety standard is needed to address an unreasonable risk of injury associated with blade contact from table saws.

Much has been done to improve the safety of art materials since the passage of the Labeling of Hazardous Art Materials Act (LHAMA) in 1988. Even so, arts and crafts materials can pose hazards. The act requires that art materials containing chemicals that can cause chronic health effects with long-term exposure be labeled to inform the user of those potential long-term effects. Examples are chemicals that are potentially carcinogenic (cancer-causing), neurotoxic (toxic to the nervous system), or teratogenic (causing birth defects). Nontoxic products are labeled "Conforms with ASTM D-4263." Read the labels on paint tubes, glues, pastels, and other art materials to find out if they present any dangers from long-term use.

RECREATION

Older people are also a growing proportion of all-terrain vehicle (ATV) operators. A review of 6,308 ATV-related traumas reported to the National Trauma Data Bank during the period 1989–2003 showed that being older than 60 years was associated with significantly longer length of hospital stay, greater number of intensive care unit days, and increased risk of dying. About 10 percent of consumer product–related deaths in the age group 65 and older reported in 2009 involved ATVs. These vehicles can be powerful and difficult to control, and they require good balance, which many older persons no longer have. Rollover incidents are relatively common. If, despite the hazards, you decide you want to operate an ATV, get training from a licensed dealer, and always wear a helmet. Know the terrain you will be negotiating, and respect the vehicle's power.

The importance of wearing a helmet is underscored by a Consumer Product Safety Commission study reporting that Baby Boomers who died from head injuries related to bicycle accidents were twice as likely to die from their injury as children who rode bikes. We correctly take action to protect the young from head injury, but their grandparents need head protection too.

8

ALL AROUND THE HOUSE

So far in this book I have talked about specific types of injuries and how and where they are most likely to happen. In the first part of this chapter I change the perspective; I start with the environment and discuss hazards and injuries by location—room by room. You can use the information to check for hazards in every room in your home or that of someone about whom you are concerned. Much of the information will sound familiar. If you are concerned about someone who has Alzheimer's disease or a related dementia or suffers from cognitive impairment of any kind, take note of the additional safety measures described for them, which are recommended by the National Institute on Aging.

The second part of this chapter describes the range of assistive and safety devices that are available for use in and around the home. Assistive devices are tools to help make your life easier. For example, to assist people with vision loss, there are phones with large numbers. Safety devices help reduce the risk of injury. For example, a device called a mixing valve controls the temperature of water delivered at a faucet to minimize the risk for scalds.

HOME REVIEW, ROOM BY ROOM

The Kitchen

The key safety concerns in the kitchen are falls, burns, and food-borne illness. To prevent falls in the kitchen, take a look at how cabinets are

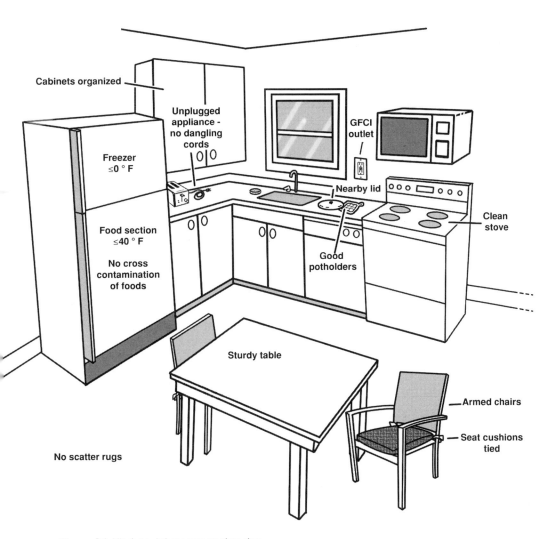

Figure 8.1. Kitchen: injury prevention tips

organized and decide if rearranging them would make it easier to reach everyday items without using a step stool. Do you have or need reaching tools (see Figure 8.3)? Check out table and chair design and placement, and look at the flooring. To prevent burns, examine the stove, the oven, the microwave, and countertop cooking appliances like toasters, toaster ovens, and coffee pots. Preventing food-borne illness involves some simple steps like checking the fridge for correct temperatures and spoiled foods, and reviewing good food wrapping and separating techniques. It also means checking non-refrigerated foods: discard any bulging cans and any dry goods (like flour and sugar) that have been infested with or contaminated by bugs, worms, or other critters, or contaminated by droppings from these pests.

PREVENTING FALLS

Start with the kitchen cabinets. Are the dishes and glassware used most often located within easy reach? Are the foods used most often within easy reach? Would grouping the foods by type make sense, for example, all cereal products together, or grouping by meal, for example, oatmeal, breakfast bars, teas, and coffee together? There is no one right way. What matters is arranging foods and plates and cutlery so you can get what you need easily and without climbing.

How do you reach things that are out of arm's reach? A low stool with no hand support may or may not offer enough stability. A kitchen stool (like a barstool) or chair is not a good option, because the step height is too high (it's awkward and unsafe to climb up onto a barstool or chair). Also, a chair or tall stool may be unstable; the legs may be uneven, causing it to wobble. When you need climbing help, you should use a sturdy step stool that has a handrail running along the sides and extending vertically to create a handle to hold on to while

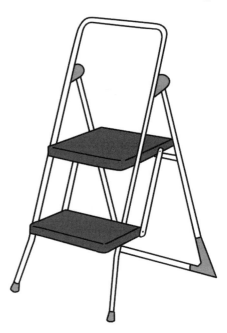

Figure 8.2. Well-designed step stool

you use the stool (Figure 8.2). If something is positioned just a little bit out of reach, a reaching tool may be useful (Figure 8.3).

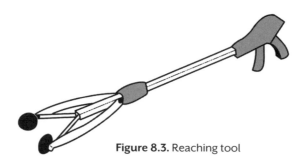

Figure 8.3. Reaching tool

Do the kitchen chairs have arms? Arms can help people get into or out of chairs. If the chairs have removable cushions, be sure they are securely in place, either held by ties to the back of the chair or kept in place by a nonslip surface on the bottom of the cushion. Slippery, unsecured cushions can slide off a chair and take with them the person who is trying to sit down or get up. Does the kitchen table have four legs or is it a pedestal table, with a center support? Pedestal tables can be unstable; if someone leans heavily on one edge, for instance when rising from a chair, a center-support table can tip over.

Next, take a look at the floor. Are there scatter rugs? It's best to remove all scatter rugs. Alternatively, place a foam nonslip pad underneath rugs. Clean up any spills *right away*; it is easy to get distracted when you are busy, and a wet floor is an invitation to fall. Have paper towels handy for cleaning up spills. Don't wax floors, because waxing makes them slippery. If you expect to be in the kitchen during the night, install a night light or leave a low-level light on.

PREVENTING BURNS

Let's start with the stove. *Stay with food while it's cooking.* Forgotten items on the stovetop are a leading cause of house fires. Be prepared and keep a pot cover handy in case of a stovetop fire. When you are cooking, wear clothing that has snug fitting or short sleeves, rather than loose, flowing, or dangling sleeves. Clean the stovetop after use to prevent grease buildup, because grease can catch fire.

Keep several good potholders on hand, not frayed or thin ones. Because containers and foods can heat unevenly in the microwave, and because some containers get hot, don't just grab an item from the microwave without first testing how hot it is to the touch. Use potholders, when needed, to take foods from the microwave, and use care to avoid spilling hot foods or liquids as you carry them from the microwave. If you know that you have lost sensitivity in your fingers, always use potholders when handling anything that might be hot. An extra second or two isn't much to spend to avoid a burn.

Unplug electrical countertop appliances after use. Check to be sure the cords of countertop appliances do not hang over the counter edge, both when appliances are plugged in and when they are unplugged. An inadvertent tug on a dangling cord can bring down an appliance and its hot contents. To reduce the risk of shock, upgrade to GFCI-equipped outlets if there are none. GFCIs (ground fault circuit interrupters), discussed in Chapter 3, should be used wherever water is used nearby.

Never cook while using medical oxygen.

PREVENTING FOOD POISONING

First to the fridge! Make sure the refrigerator compartment is set to 40°F or colder and that the freezer compartment is set to 0°F or colder. A refrigerator thermometer, carried by most supermarkets, will help you check the temperature. Go through the contents of the refrigerator, checking for leaky wrappings, items that are past their expiration dates, spoiled foods, and cross-contamination. Cross-contamination can occur when uncooked foods, especially raw meats, come into contact with ready-to-eat foods, that is, foods like fruit or salad that will not be cooked before they are consumed. Cross-contamination can happen during food preparation or in the fridge when food is not wrapped and sealed properly. Rewrap foods as necessary and discard outdated and spoiled foods. (Chapter 4 covers food safety in detail.) If necessary, clean the fridge, using a solution of baking soda and warm water on inside surfaces, and washing removable bins and shelving in warm soapy water.

Then review non-refrigerated foods, discarding products with evidence of contamination or spoilage. Check the dates on canned goods. You might want to rearrange canned goods so that you are sure to consume those with the nearest best-by dates first.

CONSIDERATIONS FOR PEOPLE WITH DEMENTIA

If a person in the house has Alzheimer's or another dementia, consider these additional safety precautions for the kitchen:

- Cover or remove knobs from the stove or install an automatic shut-off switch. Safety devices made to protect children usually work to protect adults with dementia.

- Install childproof door latches on storage cabinets, "junk drawers," and drawers containing breakable or dangerous items, like skewers. Be aware that a person with dementia may eat small items such as matches, hardware, and erasers, not understanding what they are.

- Lock away all household cleaning products, knives, scissors, blades, small appliances, and anything valuable.

- If drugs are kept in the kitchen, store all drugs, whether prescription or nonprescription, in a locked cabinet. If you keep alcoholic beverages in the house, they should also be behind a locked door.

- Remove from the house entirely any artificial fruits or vegetables and food-shaped kitchen magnets. A person with dementia may not be able to recognize that they aren't edible. Eating magnets can be particularly dangerous.

- Insert a drain trap in the kitchen sink to catch anything that may otherwise become lost or clog the plumbing.

- Disconnect the garbage disposal. People with Alzheimer's or dementia may place objects or their own hands in the disposal.

The Bedroom

The key concerns in the bedroom are falls and burns from heat sources, like space heaters and heating pads. For people who use bed rails (see Chapter 5), there is the additional concern for suffocation and strangulation, although these injuries are rare.

PREVENTING FALLS

Remove scatter rugs or place a nonskid pad underneath them. Consider installing wall-to-wall carpeting in the bedroom. Use sheets and blankets that fit the bed, and avoid silky-textured sheets, bedspreads, and quilts, which are slippery and can shift and become a tripping hazard or cause a person to slide onto the floor when trying to sit on or get off the bed. Make up the bed soon after getting up.

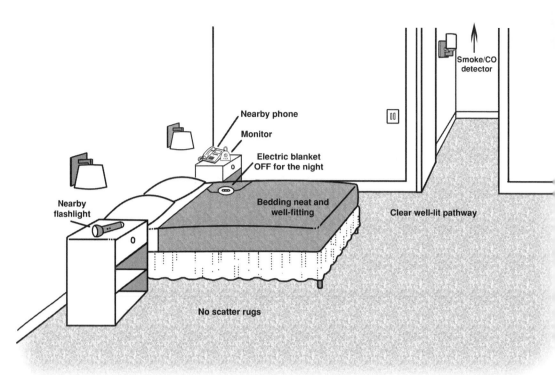

Figure 8.4. Bedroom: injury prevention tips

Remove tripping hazards, such as electrical cords, newspapers on the floor, and shoes left lying around. Create a clear, well-lit path from the bedroom to the bathroom and down any adjoining hallway. Install night lights that automatically come on in the dark and turn off at daylight. Keep a working flashlight on or in a nightstand.

If you live with someone who needs supervision and does not sleep in the same room with you, consider using an intercom device (such as a nursery monitor) to alert you to any noises indicating falls or a need for help during the night. Keep a telephone by the bed.

PREVENTING BURNS

If you use a portable electric or fuel-burning space heater, be sure it is at least three feet away from fabric or any other material that might burn. Fuel-burning heaters (for example kerosene or propane heaters) are not recommended for bedrooms because they have an open flame and generate carbon monoxide. Regardless of where electric or fuel-burning heaters might be in a house, it is wise to put them out before going to bed. Doing so prevents not only burns and fires but potential carbon monoxide poisoning. If a person has Alzheimer's or another dementia, remove portable space heaters from the person's room.

Keep the settings on electric mattress pads, electric blankets, and heating pads low when in use, and turn them off for the night just before you get into bed. It's too easy to fall asleep and forget to turn these products off. Some but not all such products have automatic shut-offs.

Never smoke in bed. If a person with dementia smokes in the house, check upholstered chairs where the person has been sitting for smoldering cigarette butts and warm ashes, and if you can, make smoking in the bedroom off limits for that person.

OTHER RISKS

If you are considering using a hospital-type bed with rails and/or wheels, read the Food and Drug Administration's up-to-date safety information at www.fda.gov for entrapment prevention. At the time of publication, the direct link was: http://www.fda.gov/Medical Devices/DeviceRegulationandGuidance/GuidanceDocuments/ucm 072662.htm.

Also see Chapter 5, Figure 1, which illustrates the potential bed rail entrapment locations.

The Bathroom

The key concerns in the bathroom are falls, scalds, drowning, and electrocution. The key preventives are some strategically placed safety and assistive devices, increased hazard awareness, and monitoring of persons who need supervision. Chapters 2 and 3 have some additional tips.

PREVENTING FALLS

Install grab bars in the tub and shower and wherever they will be helpful with maintaining balance while standing and while changing position between sitting and standing. A grab bar in contrasting color to the wall is easier to see than one that matches the wall. If standing in the shower is not an ideal option, use a plastic shower stool. A handheld shower head makes bathing easier for both standing and seated positions.

The height of the step into the shower or tub should be easy to navigate. Consider low-edged alternatives to traditional bathtubs and edgeless entries for showers.

Use an elevated toilet seat if a household member has trouble getting up and down from the toilet, because a higher toilet seat will make this process easier. Many seats—elevated or not—are equipped with handrails. If your toilet seat does not have handrails, install grab bars beside the toilet, because support is always welcome. *Towel racks are not grab bars.* They are not designed to support an adult's weight and can be pulled right out of the wall.

Use washable wall-to-wall bathroom carpeting or nonskid mats at the sink and tub to prevent slipping on wet tile floors. If the shower or tub does not have a nonslip surface, use a nonskid mat there as well.

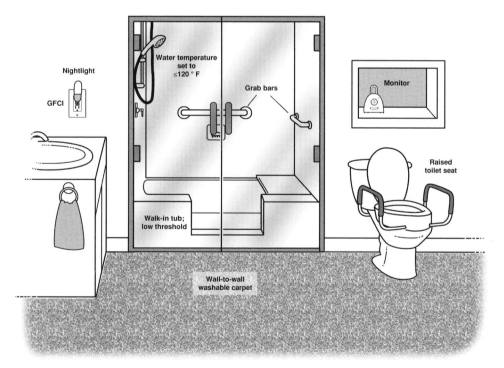

Figure 8.5. Bathroom: injury prevention tips

Install night lights both inside the bathroom and along the path to the bathroom.

Consider using an intercom device (such as a nursery monitor), so that you can be alerted if someone falls or needs help.

PREVENTING SCALDS

Adjust the water heater setting to 120°F. If the water heater has a text indicator (warm to hot) instead of numbers, you can test the water at the bathroom faucet using an instant-read cooking or bathwater thermometer and make adjustments to the water heater dial as needed. Water at 130°F will scald instantly. Consider having a plumber install mixing valves in the shower, tub, and sink to maintain a safe water temperature at the faucet. Consider covering the faucet handles so that a person with dementia can't turn on the hot water and get scalded (this approach is often recommended for bathing young children). Monitoring such persons while they bathe is a wise precaution.

PREVENTING DROWNING AND ELECTROCUTION

Drowning can be a risk for all elderly people, but if someone has a heart condition, extra care should be taken during tub bathing. Stay with the person or just outside the bathroom, engaged in conversation with the person.

To avoid electrocution in the bathroom, never use or allow others to use any electrical appliance while someone is in the bath or shower. Unplug electrical appliances after use; a plugged in appliance in the "off" position still conducts electricity! Put hairdryers and other electrical appliances away when you are done; don't leave them lying by the sink. Be sure that outlets around the sink are equipped with GFCIs (ground fault circuit interrupters) (see Chapter 3).

If a person with Alzheimer's or other dementia lives in the house, remove portable electrical appliances from the bathroom and cover electrical outlets to reduce the risk of electrocution. If men use electric razors, have them shave outside the bathroom, away from water. To prevent poisoning, remove cleaning products from under the bathroom sink or lock them away.

Finally, remove or disable the lock on the bathroom door so that if someone inside needs assistance, help will not be locked out.

The Living Room

The key concerns in the living room are falls and fire. To prevent falls, remove tripping hazards and glass coffee tables. To prevent fire, minimize the use of extension cords, be vigilant when using candles, and control fires in fireplaces and woodstoves.

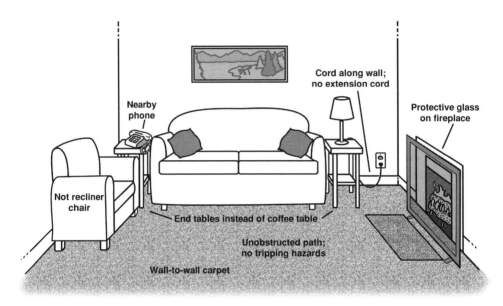

Figure 8.6. Living room: injury prevention tips

PREVENTING FALLS

Remove scatter rugs, runners, and throw rugs, or use nonslip pads under them. Repair or replace worn carpet. Clear all pathways of electrical cords, and make sure cords run along the wall and not under carpeting. If there is a telephone other than a cell phone, put it in a convenient place and make sure its cords are not in the walking path. Set the answering machine to respond after the least number of rings. This way you can be sure that the call will be promptly answered, and you will not be tempted to get up and race to answer a phone that keeps ringing.

Choose chairs that are easy to get into and out of. Recliners are not recommended for elderly persons, because they are not easy to get into or out of. Arrange furniture so that walking does not pose the challenge of an obstacle course, and keep floors clear of clutter. A magazine on the floor can cause someone who steps on it to slip and fall. Look around to see what you might land on if you did fall. Install protective caps on the corners of coffee tables to prevent or minimize fall-related injuries. Replace glass-topped coffee tables with tables made of other material; if a person falls onto a glass table, there is the possibility for a severe laceration from broken glass. For that reason and for ease of movement, you may wish to opt for end tables instead of a coffee table.

To reduce the risk of someone's walking into or through glass, place decals at eye level on any sliding glass doors, picture windows, and furniture with large glass panels, so people can easily see and recognize the glass pane.

PREVENTING FIRES

Put out candles when you leave a room. Do not have candles burning in several rooms simultaneously. Monitor fires in fireplaces and woodstoves. Never use an accelerant (a flammable liquid) to start or fuel a fire; use only the intended fuel (wood) and newspaper and kindling or a commercial starter log to get a fire going.

Do not leave a person who has dementia alone with an open fire in a fireplace. Consider alternative heating sources. Most fireplaces (including gas ones) and space heaters can get very hot, posing a burn hazard, so consider a protective guard. Do not leave matches or cigarette lighters sitting out in view of persons with dementia.

The Laundry Room

The key concern in the laundry is for people with dementia. The best way to prevent injuries is to keep such persons away from laundry facilities. Keep the door to the laundry room locked if possible. Lock all laundry products, including laundry pods, in a cabinet. Laundry pods are individually wrapped single-use detergent packets that are colorful and may resemble candy. Children have eaten these pods, thinking they were candy. An adult with cognitive limitations could make the same mistake. Remove large knobs from the washer and dryer if the person with dementia tampers with machinery. Close and latch the doors and lids to the washer and dryer to prevent objects from being placed in the machines. Child safety locks are available for washers and dryers.

The Garage, Shed, and Basement

The key concerns in these areas are carbon monoxide (CO) poisoning, fires, and tool-related lacerations or amputations.

PREVENTING CARBON MONOXIDE AND OTHER POISONINGS

Never run a generator indoors or in a garage. Generators must be placed outdoors, well away from doors and windows to the home. Store all potentially toxic products (fertilizers, paints, cleaners, etc.) in their original containers and keep them well sealed. See Chapter 4 for further information.

PREVENTING FIRES

Keep flammable materials, such as paint thinner and glues, tightly sealed. Store them well away from appliances that have a pilot light, preferably in a shed or out building. Never store gasoline in the basement or garage. Always store gasoline in a shed or out house not connected to your main home. See Chapter 3 for much more information about fire prevention.

CONSIDERATIONS FOR PEOPLE WITH DEMENTIA

Lock all garages, sheds, and basements if possible. Within these places, keep all potentially dangerous items, such as tools (power and manual), tackle, machines, and sporting equipment either locked away in cabinets or in appropriate boxes or cases. Keep all toxic materials, such as paint, fertilizers, and cleaning supplies, out of view. Either put them in a high place or lock them in a cabinet.

Secure and lock all motor vehicles. Consider covering vehicles, including bicycles, that are not frequently used. This may reduce a cognitively impaired person's thoughts of leaving.

If the person is permitted in the garage, shed, or basement, accompany him or her, and make sure that the area is well lit and that stairs have a handrail. Keep walkways clear of debris and clutter.

Throughout the Home

The following reminders for general safety improvement throughout the home focus on the added safety provided by adequate lighting, working alarm systems, knowing what to do in an emergency, and having an exit plan in case of fire.

Make sure that hallways and stairways are well lit. Install lighting both at the top and at the bottom of stairs and at both ends of hallways. Check all rooms for adequate lighting.

Ideally, stairways will have two handrails, but all stairways should have at least one handrail that extends beyond the first and last steps. Always hold the handrail when going up or down stairs. If possible, stairways should be carpeted or have safety grip strips.

Avoid clutter, which can create a tripping hazard, distraction, and confusion. Throw out or recycle newspapers and magazines regularly. Keep all walking areas free of furniture.

Install smoke alarms and carbon monoxide detectors near all sleeping areas on all levels of the home. Check that they are in working order and at least twice a year—for instance, when you change the clocks for Daylight Saving Time and back again—change the batteries in the alarms. Schedule a visit by a representative from your local fire department to inspect your home to be sure it meets local safety codes for these devices.

Do not allow smoking around home-use oxygen. The person wearing the oxygen should keep at least ten feet away from any flame or heat source. Never cook while using oxygen. Post a sign on the door or window visible to those entering indicating that oxygen is in use and that smoking, sparks, and open flame are prohibited.

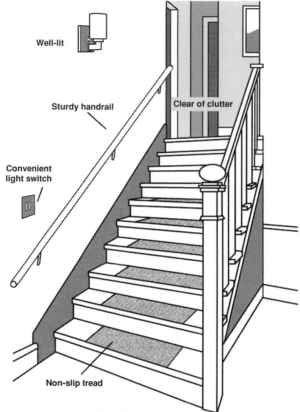

Well-lit

Sturdy handrail

Clear of clutter

Convenient
light switch

Non-slip tread

Figure 8.7. Stairway: injury prevention tips

Display emergency numbers and your home address near all telephones.
The number to call for fire and ambulance is 911. The number to call
for poison centers is 800-222-1222.

Create a fire escape plan and practice it. (See Chapter 3.)

Remove all poisonous plants from the home. Check with local nurs-
eries or poison control centers for a list of house plants that if eaten
or chewed on would make a person sick.

CONSIDERATIONS FOR PEOPLE WITH DEMENTIA

Because persons with dementia may not be able to take telephone
messages and can become victims of telephone exploitation, turn
telephone ringers off or set them to low if the person will be home
alone. Put all portable phones and cell phones and equipment in

a safe place so they will not be easily lost. Hide a spare house key outside, in case the ill person locks you out of the house.

Keep all medications (prescription and over-the-counter) in a locked drawer or cabinet. Keep thin plastic bags (for example dry cleaning bags) out of reach because they could pose a suffocation hazard.

Keep fish tanks out of reach. The combination of glass, water, electrical pumps, and potentially poisonous aquatic life could be harmful to a curious person with Alzheimer's.

While we are discussing general home safety, gun storage requires special attention. More older persons than younger persons own a gun. A 2004 survey showed that 27 percent of those 65 and older personally owned a firearm. That means that quite a few more people live in a home that has a gun in it. In 2011, 37.2 percent of Americans aged 65 or older lived in a home with a firearm.

Fear of crime is a driving factor in gun ownership among the elderly, in spite of the fact that they are far less likely than are younger people to be to victims of violent crime. Ironically, among older people, gun ownership increases the risk of violent death, including suicide and homicide-suicide. A gun is the most common means of suicide in the United States, and the rates of firearm suicide are highest among people 75 or older. Suicide in this group is less likely to be related to mental health problems and more likely to be related to physical health. According to 2010 data from the National Violent Death Reporting System, with sixteen states reporting, in 93 percent of homicide-suicide cases in which a victim was 65 or older, an intimate partner was involved. In some of these cases, a man killed his wife or partner, and then himself, in a "mercy killing" to end a long illness.

For people with Alzheimer's or other dementia, gun ownership or access is particularly problematic. Memory loss, confusion, aggressive behavior, and personality changes put them, and their caretakers, at great risk. The most effective measure to keep all persons safe is to remove all guns and other weapons from the home. If a person chooses to keep a firearm in the home, the gun must be stored safely. Safe gun storage means keeping guns and ammunition separate; place the *unloaded* gun in a locked box, out of sight, and store ammunition in another locked box separate from the gun.

Approaches to the House

As with the interior of the home, falls are the key concern as one approaches the exterior of a house. To prevent such falls, make sure that exterior steps are solid, and minimize slippery, rocky, or uneven pavement. Sufficient lighting is also essential.

Eliminate uneven outside surfaces and clear walkways of hoses and other tripping hazards. Keep hoses on a hose wheel or rack. Prune bushes and foliage well away from walkways and doorways. Steps should be in good repair, easily negotiated, and equipped with a handrail. Textured steps help prevent falls in wet or icy weather. For added visibility of steps, mark the edges with bright or reflective tape or paint.

Make sure outside lighting is adequate. Light sensors that turn on lights automatically as you approach the house may be useful. They also may be used in other parts of the home. Photosensitive lights turn on automatically when it gets dark.

Placing a chair near the door you usually use can be helpful. You may be tired from an outing or you may be juggling bundles as you return home. In either case, it is nice to have a place to rest right as you get inside. If there is space, place a seat or bench near the entry door so you can set packages down—or sit down yourself, if you need to—as soon as you get home. Such an arrangement enhances safety as well as comfort.

Restrict access to a backyard swimming pool, spa, or hot tub by surrounding it on all four sides with fencing equipped with a self-latching gate that opens outward. Check your local building codes for requirements. Adequate fencing also serves to prevent access by neighborhood toddlers and young children, who are at high risk of drowning in backyard pools. If a side of the house is used to complete the fourth side of fencing (as shown in the illustration), install window and door alarms to alert you when someone exits the house into the pool area. When the pool is not in use, cover it with a safety cover. When it is in use, supervise closely.

In addition, if a person in the home has Alzheimer's or another dementia, remove the fuel source and fire starters from any backyard grills when not in use and supervise use when the person is present.

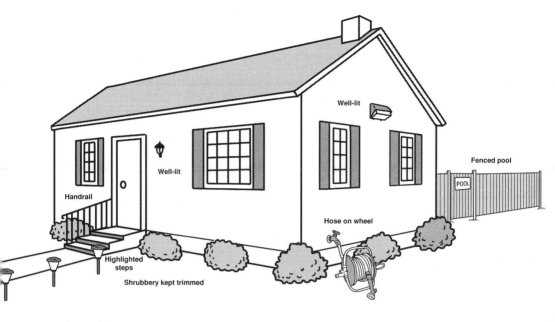

Figure 8.8. Exterior: injury prevention tips

ASSISTIVE AND SAFETY DEVICES

Many assistive devices not only assist—they also increase safety. A device that allows you to reach and retrieve objects from high shelves, for example, both helps you quickly reach something you want and keeps you from climbing onto a chair or stretching in a way that throws you off balance. There are also devices designed specifically to increase safety, for example fall prevention devices. The assistive devices described below are arranged by the sense that they help (hearing, vision, and so on). The safety devices are categorized by the hazard they help avoid. These lists are by no means exhaustive, as the number and types of products on the market are extensive and growing, but they will give you an idea of the kinds of products available. When you consider the options of assistive technology, it could be useful to separate the options into high-tech and low-tech solutions. High-tech devices tend to be more expensive but may be able to assist with many different needs. Low-tech equipment is usually cheaper but less adaptable for multiple purposes.

Before purchasing any assistive technology, older adults should carefully evaluate their needs. A team approach is often most helpful. For example, an older person who has trouble communicating or is hard of hearing should consult with his or her audiology specialist, a speech-language therapist, and family and friends. Together, this team of people can identify the problem more precisely and can help select the most effective devices available at the lowest cost. A professional member of the team, such as the audiology specialist, can also educate and coach the older person and other family members in how to use the devices properly.

These recommendations are based on information from MedlinePlus (nlm.nih.gov/medlineplus/assistivedevices.html), a plain-language medical website for patients and their families and friends.

Hearing

Assistive listening devices (ALDs) are intended to assist people with hearing loss. They typically work by magnifying sounds, selectively directing sounds to the person, or replacing a sound with a visual or tactile stimulus. Examples of common products include alarm clocks and watches that either are very loud or vibrate at the set time, door bells that trigger a light inside the home to come on, smoke and carbon monoxide alarms that either sound at a specific pitch the person can hear or send out a light signal, phones equipped with TTY, which is a text telephone or teleprinter specifically designed for text communication over a public telephone network, captioned telephones, which utilize speech recognition technology to display a text version of the ongoing conversation, and answering machines that make messages louder and slower.

Other assistive hearing devices include looping systems, telecoils, TV ears, and Bluetooth technology. Looping systems generate a magnetic signal and are designed to work with public address systems in places like auditoriums and churches. Looped rooms are wired so that any sound from a public address speaker goes directly to headphones a listener puts on or directly to a person's hearing aids if they are equipped with a telecoil, also known as a T-coil. The loop system eliminates the interference from background sounds, so the listener hears the selected sound with great clarity.

A telecoil, or T-coil, is a device that can be incorporated into a hearing aid. It is a tiny coil of wire around a core that responds to changes in the magnetic field. T-coils are available for most behind-the-ear hearing aids and for some in-the-ear hearing aids. Your audiologist can help you learn about and consider these devices. (Audiology and hearing aids are discussed in Chapter 9.)

"TV ears" and other wireless TV listening devices enable people with a hearing loss to listen to television at a volume comfortable for them without having to make the volume uncomfortably loud for other people. These devices consist of a transmitter connected to the television and a receiver built into wireless headphones the person wears. The person controls the volume from the headset.

Bluetooth technology was invented by the Swedish company Ericsson. The inventors wanted to use Bluetooth as a collaborative tool to connect multiple electronic devices so as to share information quickly over the air. In 1998, a group of companies formed the Bluetooth Special Interest Group, an organization in which no one individual "owns" Bluetooth technology and all members work together to further develop and maintain the technology. Bluetooth technology for hearing assistance allows you to connect (called "pairing") wirelessly, via a device called a "streamer," to your phone, television, or other audio device, and receive exceptionally clear sounds directly to your hearing aids.

Vision

Low vision, defined as a level of vision of 20/70 or worse that cannot be corrected with conventional glasses, is not a normal part of aging, but it does primarily affect the elderly. Most people develop low vision because of eye diseases. Among the aging population, common causes of low vision are macular degeneration, glaucoma, and diabetic retinopathy. People with these eye diseases have some useful sight, but their vision loss affects their ability to read, drive, and perform other daily activities. For example, a person with low vision may not recognize images at a distance or may not be able to differentiate colors of similar tones. (See Chapter 1 for a description and illustration of the effects on vision of these conditions.) There are many tools available to assist people with low vision. Many books and other materials are published in large print versions. A wide variety of magnifiers is available: handheld magnifiers,

magnifiers that clip to your eyeglasses or fit over your head, desktop magnifiers that project the text onto a screen, video magnifiers (closed circuit TVs), software that magnifies computer images, and specialized camera products that send images to a viewing screen or to your computer. Other products communicate verbally. These include products that scan text and read it back to you; talking clocks, wristwatches, and calculators; and talking global positioning system (GPS) devices that tell you the names of streets, intersections, and landmarks as you walk or ride along.

Balance

Many products help with balance. As discussed in Chapter 2, although people using walkers and canes face particular risks of falling, these assistive devices allow people to remain mobile, which is extremely important to a person's mental and physical health. The key to safer use of these aids is learning how to use them correctly. They must also fit you in terms of height and comfort. If you are buying one of these products on your own (rather than getting one directly from a health care professional or facility), get a knowledgeable person from a medical supply store to assist you with both the fit and instructions on how to use it properly.

Grab bars provide assistance, whether you are standing still or transitioning between standing and sitting. They can be installed in the shower or tub, and on any wall. They are an easy and effective aid. Because bathrooms present numerous challenges to balance, you may have to consider making some structural changes in your bathroom in addition to installing grab bars. Stepping into a shower or tub may once have been easy, but the step height may now be a bit challenging—and dangerous, if it throws you off balance. You can buy bathtub door inserts that fit onto your existing tub, or you can buy a walk-in tub. These devices eliminate the need to step over a high side. For a less costly and simpler solution, you can buy a transfer bench, which straddles the tub. You sit down on the side of the bench outside of the tub, then slide over to the portion inside the tub. Various designs are available.

You can also buy shower stalls that are flush with the floor or have only a slight (half-inch or so) rise to floor level, for easy entry. These stalls make it easy for someone in a wheelchair to use the shower. Once in the shower or tub, bath seats can be very useful. Handheld shower heads are a better option than fixed shower heads, which pour water from overhead onto the person.

Toilet seat height can be a problem. A higher seat is easier to get down to and up from. You can have a taller toilet installed, but an easier, cheaper solution is to buy a raised toilet seat that fits onto the toilet you already have. Styles with arms offer added balance support.

Strength and Flexibility

Strength assistance products abound. They include aids for cooking, eating, gardening, grooming and more. Examples include jar openers, angled kitchen and garden utensils that keep your wrist in a neutral position, doorknob covers that help with gripping and twisting, and easy-grip scissors. There are also exercise products designed to strengthen hand grip.

Fine motor skill and flexibility aids help with getting dressed. There are zipper pulls, button hooks, dressing sticks, sock aids, long-handled shoehorns, and so on. In addition, there is adaptive clothing, specifically designed to make dressing easier for yourself or for the person helping someone get dressed. Examples include pants with long zippers extending down the legs on both sides, shoes with Velcro® instead of laces, and tops that open in the back, allowing the person to easily put both arms into sleeves simultaneously.

Fall Prevention

Fall prevention aids include socks with textured grippers on the bottoms, nonslip mats, and slip-resistant stair and floor tape. Tools like reach bars (see Figure 8.3) that help you to reach items from a standing or seated position rather than by climbing reduce the chances of falling off step stools or chairs and of overextending your reach and losing your balance.

Chapter 5 discusses the pros and cons of using bed rails to prevent falls from beds.

Scald Prevention

Mixing valves, installed by a plumber, ensure that the temperature of the water delivered at the faucet is not hot enough to scald. This solution takes away the danger of a surge of hot water and of mistakenly turning on excessively hot water. Faucet handle covers, which are often used to protect children, also work for older adults with dementia.

Poison Prevention

Keeping your medications organized will reduce the chances of overdosing or underdosing. Pill organizers are readily available at pharmacies, as are dosage dispensers (for example, for a liquid drug) and pill cutters. If a person cannot safely take medications on his or her own, buy a locking cabinet to keep the medications in; this will avoid the dangers posed by unsupervised access.

9

SEEING THE DOCTOR

One way to reduce the risk of injury is to stay as healthy as you can. We have discussed the injury preventive benefits of exercise, good nutrition, hearing and vision care, and attention to medication regimens. Regular checkups with your doctor also help keep you strong and healthy. A key component of any visit to a doctor is understanding what happened during the visit. Understanding what your doctor tells you and what you read about your health is called "health literacy." The term "health literacy" is defined as "the degree to which individuals have the capacity to obtain, process, and understand basic health information and services needed to make appropriate health or medical decisions." To get an idea of your level of health literacy, think about a recent visit you have had with a doctor and ask yourself the following questions:

- Did I come away from the visit with a thorough understanding of what went on? Did I ask questions about anything I did not fully understand? (The answer to these questions should be yes.)

- Did I agree for the sake of agreeing, without having a clear understanding of what I was agreeing with? (The answer should be no.)

- Could I hear everything the doctor said, or did I "fill in" with what I thought he meant when I could not make out what was being said? (You should be able to hear what your doctor is saying and say so if you can't.)

- Was I able to accurately answer questions about myself? Did I understand the forms I was asked to fill out? (The answers should be yes.)

The first part of this chapter explains how to become more health literate and how to get the most from your doctor visits. The second part of the chapter further explores treatment of four specific areas of health: hearing, vision, feet, and teeth. Making the most of the assistance available in these areas of health care will help you stay active and healthy longer.

HEALTH LITERACY AND COMMUNICATION

Health literacy gives you the tools to make good health decisions. An astonishing 40 percent of the U.S. population is affected by low health literacy; the adults most vulnerable to health illiteracy are older people, people with limited English-language proficiency, poor people, homeless people, and people with less education. People with low health literacy may have difficulty with a number of tasks that are crucial for good health, such as:

understanding and following directions for taking medications

reading a nutrition label

asking questions of doctors

sharing their medical history with health care providers

completing health information forms

understanding preventive care

In contrast, people with good health literacy can find information from books, the Internet, and elsewhere; read and understand information; read prescription bottles; take medications correctly; follow complex instructions, such as the preparation needed for a colonoscopy; make and keep appointments more successfully; and complete health information forms, such as a family medical history.

Low health literacy puts people at risk for failing to seek out and receive good health care, and it puts people's safety at risk because they lack a good understanding of what they should do about their health. For example, many people who are trying to conserve their funds decide to make their medication go further by cutting their pills in half—without understanding how the reduced drug dosage may affect their health.

The following additional examples highlight some common areas of misunderstanding about medicine which can lead to errors.

DO YOU REALLY UNDERSTAND THE DOSAGE SCHEDULE?

For example, if the instructions for a medication say to take it every four hours, do you need to get up in the middle of the night to stay on schedule or should you take the medicine only during the hours you are awake? (You should ask the doctor or pharmacist.)

ARE YOU ABLE TO CALIBRATE YOUR GLUCOSE METER CORRECTLY?

If you are a diabetic who should be checking your blood sugar levels, do you follow the instructions to ensure that the glucose meter is reading accurately, or do you skip that step and assume the meter is correct? (Calibrating the glucose meter makes it an accurate tool; without calibration, it is much less useful or possibly useless.)

DO YOU GET FLU SHOTS AND TAKE ADVANTAGE OF OTHER PREVENTIVE MEASURES?

Do you know where to get influenza and other vaccines? Do you know which vaccinations you should get? (Flu shots and other vaccines can ward off illnesses that in some cases may even be fatal. Your doctor, health clinic, and pharmacy can help.)

DO YOU UTILIZE THE HOSPITAL EMERGENCY ROOM AS YOUR "DOCTOR"?

Do you have a relationship with a doctor from whom you can seek treatment guidance? (Regularly seeing and communicating with a doctor who knows you may result in better health outcomes.)

There is a lot of information to process when we interact with the health care system. Having a friend or family member go with you to a doctor's appointment, especially if you are sick at the time, is a good way to improve your health literacy. For one thing, we all have more trouble paying attention and taking in information when we are sick, stressed, tired, anxious, or depressed. Your companion—it can be a son or daughter, a relative, or a friend—can take notes, help you remember events and dates, help you ask questions, and generally be your advocate. Your companion should be a person who has good cognitive skills and is alert enough to act as a second pair of ears and eyes for you. After the appointment, your advocate can help you remember what went on at the doctor's office and be sure it is written down for your home health record.

One way the concept of health literacy is making an impact in the public arena is by placing more responsibility on the health community to improve how it delivers information. A U.S. government program called Healthy People noted that "clear, candid, accurate, culturally and linguistically competent provider-patient communication is essential for prevention, diagnosis, treatment and management of health concerns." Healthy People sets ten-year national objectives for improving the health of all Americans. The current program, Healthy People 2020, has defined more than forty areas for health objectives, including the health of older adults. One of the objectives is to increase the proportion of older adults with one or more chronic conditions who report confidence in their own ability to manage their illnesses. You can see the role of health literacy in this objective; it means that people understand how to take their medications, know how to follow dietary restrictions, adhere to exercise or rehabilitation programs, and so on. The program also provides information on a wide range of health issues written in easy-to-understand language. To access this program's website, go to www.healthypeople.gov/2020.

This improvement in how health information is delivered is an important step forward. Communication is a two-way process. Doctors need to be trained to watch for the signs of low health literacy, such as a disparity when a person claims that he or she is taking their medications correctly but the lab tests do not show the results that would be expected if this were true. If the problem is a misunderstanding on the part of the patient, the doctor must assume some responsibility for failing to communicate in a manner that the patient could comprehend. The doctor is the teacher and the patient the pupil. If the pupil is having trouble learning, it is the teacher who must try a new technique. Doctors should consider utilizing several different ways to deliver information: drawings or diagrams, videos, pamphlets or brochures, websites, storytelling, and so on. To ensure patient understanding, the doctor can ask the patient to repeat what he or she understood and should encourage the patient to ask further questions.

The patient needs to hold up the other side of the conversation. The National Patient Safety Foundation's Partnership for Clear Health Communication encourages the "Ask me 3" approach for patients: three good questions to ask every time you speak with a health professional (doctor, nurse, pharmacist, etc.):

1. What is my main problem?

2. What do I need to do?

3. Why is it important for me to do this?

These very basic questions help to focus the discussion so that you get the information you need. To learn more, go to npsf.org/askme3.

Three other good questions relate specifically to medications:

1. What is this medicine for?

2. How should I take it?

3. What should I expect from the medicine, both the benefits and side effects?

Much remains to be done to simplify our health care maze. Just consider how difficult it is to choose a health insurance plan or a prescription drug plan. Do you understand your eligibility? Once you decide on a plan, do you understand your coverage? Do you understand those explanation of benefit (EOB) letters you get?

Health literacy campaigns call for language that can be understood the first time people read or hear it, so they can find what they need, understand what they find, and use what they find to meet their needs.

YOU AND YOUR DOCTOR

Now let's examine how you can make the most of your visits to your doctor, whether he or she is your primary care physician or a specialist.

Are You Happy with Your Doctor?

Your visits to your doctor should be two-way conversations. You ought to have the opportunity to ask questions and to confirm that you understand what the doctor is saying. You ought to feel comfortable speaking about sensitive issues, and you must be able to trust in the care you are receiving. What are you looking for in a doctor? Make a list of the things that are important to you. Your list might include:

- Am I more comfortable with a man or woman doctor, or is gender not important to me?

- Do I want my doctor to be affiliated with a particular hospital?

- Do I want a doctor with an individual practice or one who is part of a group so that group partners are available for me to see as well?

- Are office hours or office location important to me?

- Do I want a doctor who speaks my native language?

- Do I want to be able to e-mail the doctor? Have a phone conversation with the doctor?

- Do I want a doctor who considers alternative or complementary forms of care, like acupuncture?

- Am I prepared to pay extra to see a doctor who is outside my insurance plan's network? HMOs (health maintenance organizations) and PPOs (preferred provider organizations) are networks of doctors. If you have one of these kinds of insurance, you may be required to see a doctor within that network or to pay extra if you wish to see one who is outside your network.

If You Decide to Find a New Doctor

Doctors understand that patients' needs change, and they understand that you must feel comfortable with your doctor. Do not decide to stay with a doctor you don't really care for because you think you might hurt his or her feelings by seeing someone else. Your care is the most important factor.

- Ask friends, relatives, and medical and health care professionals which doctors they have had good experiences with and why.

- Look online for a doctor. Go to the American Medical Association website (ama-assn.org) and click on "find a doctor."

- Check out doctors' credentials. Many libraries have directories, such as the *Directory of Physicians in the United States* and the *Official American Board of Certified Medical Specialists*. For the most convenient source, go to MedlinePlus, the National Institutes of Health's website for patients, their families, and friends: nlm.nih.gov/medlineplus/directories.html. There you will find links to various helpful directories.

- Find out if a doctor you are considering is taking new patients.

- Make sure your insurance will be accepted by the doctor's office. Find out if the doctor is accepting Medicare patients. If you are receiving Medicaid, ask if the doctor accepts it.

- Call your local or state medical society to find out if any complaints have been filed against a doctor you are considering.

- Consider setting up an appointment to "interview" the doctor. You will probably have to pay for this visit, but it will give you the best information about the doctor, his staff, and his office to help you make a decision.

Seeing a New Doctor

When you start receiving care from a different doctor, ask that your medical records be sent from your previous doctor's office *before* your first visit. It will save both you and the doctor a lot of time if he or she can review your records before seeing you. It will make you feel more relaxed if you do some advanced planning and thinking.

- How will you get to the doctor's? If you are driving, know the route and where to park once you arrive. If you are taking public transportation, know the schedule, how far you may have to walk, and where you have to wait for the bus or train.

- Bring with you a list of all the medicines (prescriptions and over-the-counter products) you are taking and perhaps even take the bottles with you. Let the doctor know of any recent changes in your medications or symptoms. One good way to keep a record of your medicines is illustrated in Table 9.1.

- Make a list of all the concerns you want to discuss with the doctor. Start with the most important concerns. If there are major stresses in your life, let the doctor know what those are. Stress is a significant factor in health. This is not complaining; the doctor needs to know these things in order to make appropriate treatment plans for you.

- When discussing treatments, ask what the options are and how the different choices could affect you and your lifestyle. Ask about risks.

- Ask about preventive measures. What can you do to avoid illness and maintain health?

- Be honest in answering the doctor when he or she asks about your lifestyle, eating and sleeping habits, smoking and drinking habits, moods, and so on. Don't report what you think the doctor wants to hear; report what's true. Your honesty will help the doctor understand you better and make appropriate treatment recommendations for you.

- If you wear glasses or hearing devices, be sure to take them with you. Many older people misunderstand medical advice because they cannot hear well. Let the doctor and the office staff know if you need to receive written materials in large print or if you need for them to speak slowly and clearly so you can understand. These requests are nothing to be embarrassed about.

Table 9.1. Example of Medicine Record

Name	What for?	Dosage	Shape and color of pill	Prescribing doctor	Date started	Date ended*
Lovastatin	Cholesterol	20 mg once at dinner	Round, pale yellow	Smith	10/20/2005	
Aspirin	Blood thinner	1 baby (81 mg) once a day	Round, pink	Smith	5/1/2009	
Calcium	Bones	500 mg twice a day	Elongated, light gray	None	4/1/2009	

*Consult with your doctor on how to stop taking any medication. Many medications will cause negative side effects if you stop taking them abruptly; your doctor will tell you how to wean yourself off them safely.

Note: Always tell your doctor about any prescription or over-the-counter medications or supplements, including herbal preparations, that you are taking, regularly or even occasionally.

- Bring someone with you—that advocate discussed earlier in this chapter. Ask him or her to take notes as you talk with the doctor; a lot of ground is covered in an initial office visit, and it is unlikely that you will remember everything that went on. If you want some time to be private between you and your doctor, let your companion know that as well.

- If you have any follow-up questions or need clarification on what the doctor said, jot down your questions and call the doctor's office.

If the Doctor Prescribes a New Medicine

It is not unusual for a new doctor to make some changes in a patient's medication regimen, either which medicines are being taken or the dosages. Talk with the doctor if you have concerns about polypharmacy, that is, taking many medications simultaneously (discussed in Chapter 2). Remember that the goal is to find the right medication for you at the right dosage and for the shortest possible duration.

These are some questions you might ask the doctor or your pharmacist about a new medicine prescribed for you. If it helps, write down the answers.

- What is the name of the medicine, and why am I taking it? Is it available and just as effective in a less expensive generic form?

- How many times a day should I take it? At what times? If the bottle says take "4 times a day," does that mean 4 times in 24 hours or 4 times during the daytime?

- Should I take the medicine with food or without? Is there anything I should not eat or drink while taking this medicine?

- What does "as needed" mean?

- When should I stop taking the medicine?

- If I forget to take my medicine, what should I do?

- What side effects can I expect? What should I do if I have a problem?

Remind your doctor about any allergies and any problems you have had with medicines, such as rashes, indigestion, dizziness, or mood changes.

HEARING HEALTH

Because good hearing and vision are critical to overall health and safety, in addition to seeing a medical doctor, you might also see a doctor of audiology for your hearing health and a doctor of optometry for your vision health. A doctor of audiology is not a medical doctor but is a specialist in diagnosing and treating hearing problems. A doctor of optometry is not a medical doctor but is a specialist in evaluating your vision and prescribing corrective lenses. Hearing and vision are so important that you should be as picky about whom you see for these services as you are about your medical doctor.

The American Speech-Language-Hearing Association recommends having your hearing checked every three years after age 50. While many people are aware that their hearing is not what it used to be, they hesitate to see a hearing specialist because they don't want to acknowledge their loss and they don't want to wear hearing aids. Often it is an exhausted family member—exhausted from repeating phrases, shouting, putting up with a loud TV, and so on—who finally convinces a person to seek help. Here are some symptoms that tell you it's time to see an audiologist.

- have trouble hearing over the telephone

- find it hard to follow conversations when two or more people are talking

- often ask people to repeat what they are saying

- need to turn up the TV volume so loud that others complain

- have a problem hearing because of background noise

- think that others are mumbling

- can't understand when women and children speak

When you make the decision to have your hearing tested, the following explanation of terms will be helpful. An *audiologist* is professionally trained and licensed by the state to measure hearing loss and to fit hearing aids. At a minimum an audiologist has a masters degree and specialized training in hearing loss; in addition, some audiologists have a doctoral degree (Au.D. or Ph.D.). As of 2011, audiologists must have a minimum of a doctoral degree to practice. The doctoral degree requires four years of academic training beyond a bachelor's degree. Coursework includes: anatomy, physiology, physics, genetics, normal and abnormal communication development, diagnosis and treatment of hearing problems, pharmacology, and ethics. Graduate programs also include supervised clinical practice.

A *hearing instrument specialist* (HIS) is someone authorized by the state to sell hearing aids. The credentials vary by state but typically involve taking a three-month class in subjects related to hearing, working as an apprentice to an already certified HIS, and passing a test about hearing aids in the state where the person is going to practice. A hearing instrument specialist is not an audiologist and does not have the academic training that an audiologist has. An HIS can "screen" for hearing loss but cannot evaluate, diagnose, or treat hearing loss. An HIS may have no education beyond high school. You are more likely to find an HIS working for a chain of retail stores that sell hearing aids, such as Costco or Miracle Ear®, whereas a doctor of audiology typically has an individual private practice, practices out of the office of an otolaryngologist (an ENT, a medical doctor who specializes in ear, nose, and throat health), or practices out of a hospital setting.

A *doctor of audiology* (Au.D.) provides individualized and continuous care of your hearing, much like your medical doctor does for your general health. For example, based on information from the American Academy of Audiology, a doctor of audiology

- uses audiometers, computers, and other devices to examine patients who have hearing, balance, or related ear problems in order to determine the extent of hearing damage and identify the underlying cause

- assesses the results of the examination and diagnoses problems

- determines and administers treatment

- fits and dispenses hearing aids

- teaches patients how to use and care for hearing aids

- counsels patients and their families on ways to listen and communicate

- can treat tinnitus (ringing or noises in the ears)

- sees patients regularly to check on hearing and balance and to continue or change the treatment plan

- keeps records on the progress of patients

Doctors of audiology measure the volume at which a person begins to hear sounds and the person's ability to distinguish between types of sounds. Before recommending treatment options, they evaluate psychological information to estimate the impact of hearing loss on a patient. They also counsel patients on other ways of coping with profound hearing loss, such as lip reading and American Sign Language.

Since balance is such a significant factor in falls (see Chapter 2), and since the balance system is closely related to the hearing system, ask your audiologist to assess your balance. This should be a routine part of your hearing evaluation.

What You Should Know about Types of Hearing Loss

Sometimes, a hearing loss can be a symptom of a medical condition. A medical examination may uncover underlying illnesses or medical problems associated with your hearing loss. The U.S. Food and Drug Administration (FDA) regards a medical evaluation in the case of hearing loss so important that it requires all hearing aid sellers to tell clients that they should receive a medical examination *before*

buying a hearing aid. The FDA also stipulates that people who decide to forego a medical evaluation before purchasing hearing aids
must sign a waiver.

There are three common types of hearing loss: conductive, sensorineural, and mixed (a combination of those other two). Conductive hearing loss involves the outer ear, the middle ear, or both.
(The human ear has three distinct sections, referred to as the outer,
middle, and inner ear.) Conductive hearing loss usually results
from a blockage by ear wax in the outer ear, a collection of fluid
in the middle ear, a punctured ear drum, or disruption of the tiny
bones (ossicles) behind the ear drum. Removal of ear wax and fluid
is often easily performed by an otolaryngologist. Other middle ear
problems may require surgery.

Sensorineural hearing loss involves damage to the inner ear. It
can be caused by age, disease, illness, noise exposure, genetics, or
exposure to certain medications (called ototoxic medications). This
type of hearing loss cannot be corrected surgically but can be corrected or helped with hearing aids. This is the most common type
of hearing loss among older people.

Mixed hearing loss may be treated by surgery, medication, hearing aids, or a combination of those treatments.

What You Should Know about Types of Hearing Aids

First, you will be amazed at the technology behind today's hearing
aids. They are smaller, smarter, and more powerful than ever. Older
generation hearing aids (based on analog technology) just made all
sounds louder; today's digital hearing aids adjust for the different
kinds of sounds and noises you hear, can be programmed for particular hearing environments (for example concerts, meetings, or
quiet time), and allow you to hear in a manner much closer to the
way people normally hear. Bluetooth technology (mentioned in
Chapter 8) allows the hearing aids to connect, via a device called a
streamer, to your phone, television, or other audio device, making
those sounds amazingly clear.

Depending on your type of hearing loss, you might be treated
with behind-the-ear aids, in-the-ear aids, or completely-in-the-
canal (deep and not visible) aids. Cochlear implants are surgically

inserted devices helpful to some people with severe hearing loss. Cochlear implants are tiny devices that are placed under the skin near the ear in a surgical operation performed by a medical doctor. Another part of the device is external and visible behind the ear. Cochlear implants deliver electrical impulses directly to the auditory nerve in the brain so that a person with certain types of deafness can hear.

Buying hearing aids online or via mail order is not recommended, because hearing aids must be custom fitted to work properly. Don't get lured by the cheaper pricing offered by those who sell hearing aids online or through the mail. The fact is that, if you have a hearing loss that causes you problems, you need a person offering you continuous care for your hearing health.

Wherever you purchase your hearing aids, ask about the trial period policy and which fees are refundable if you return the hearing aids during that period. Also ask about future service, warranty, and repair.

A Personal Story

If you are hesitating to see someone about your hearing loss, read this excerpt from a true story, as told to a doctor of audiology in 2012 and published in a local newspaper (*Old Colony Memorial*, Plymouth, MA):

> I knew I had a hearing problem, but didn't address the issue for about 15 years. . . . All that changed a month ago when I received a notice from your office about the newest technology in hearing aids. I was a little skeptical at first, but I said "go see what's new." I did and I am thankful for that. I was fitted with a demo for each ear and immediately heard the difference. My devices came in about two weeks and now I can hear things I haven't heard in a long time. I am not afraid to join conversations or talk to people in crowds. . . . It has really made a definite difference in my life. You don't really understand how hearing loss affects your life until you don't hear for a while and then suddenly are able to hear. It is truly a relief and people around you notice the difference also. I was fitted for the devices and you can hardly notice them. I'm thankful I took the step and relied on your expertise.

This person's experience is not an isolated case. People often begin to cry when they receive hearing aids and hear for the first time in a long while the sounds that were once familiar. Having one's hearing restored can be overwhelmingly beautiful and emotional.

Here is another issue that is relevant for a discussion with your audiologist. Do you have ringing or other noises in the ears? Tinnitus is the perception of sound that has no external source. Some of the common sounds people with tinnitus report hearing are ringing, roaring, hissing, humming, buzzing, and cricket-like sounds. Sounds can stay the same, change, be constant, intermittent, or be heard in one or both ears or in the head. Current theory is that tinnitus is caused by neural activity in the brain and auditory system that has been triggered by, among many possibilities, stress, diet, hearing loss, natural aging, noise exposure, head injury, infections, or side effects from medications. It can also be a sign of other health problems, such as high blood pressure or allergies, so anyone experiencing tinnitus should also consult a medical doctor.

Tinnitus sometimes gets worse over time and in other cases does not. Severe tinnitus can be disabling to some individuals and can lead to depression. Although there is no cure, there are treatments that can alleviate the severity of the condition.

VISION HEALTH

Vision care is as integral to maintaining health as we age as hearing care is. By the time most of us have reached our fifth decade, we are wearing some form of corrective lenses. As we continue to age, we may experience a specific eye disease, like glaucoma, cataracts, macular degeneration, or retinal diseases. (These eye diseases and how they affect vision are described in Chapter 1.) Some vision changes can affect one's driving: greater sensitivity to glare from oncoming vehicle lights, the sun, or even street lights; greater difficulty seeing clearly at night; having to be closer to street or traffic signs in order to read them; and taking longer to recognize familiar places.

"Low vision" is a reduction in visual acuity to 20/70 or worse that makes everyday tasks difficult. A person with low vision may find it difficult or impossible to read, write, go shopping, watch television, drive a car, or recognize faces. A deterioration of your vision doesn't mean that you have to give up certain activities; it just means you may have to find new ways to do them. (See Chapter 8 for visual assistive tools.)

The National Institute on Aging recommends that you have your vision checked every one to two years if you are 65 or older. You may see one or more specialists in getting your eyes checked. The following explanation of terms will be helpful.

An *optometrist* (doctor of optometry, O.D.) is not a medical doctor but trains for four years beyond a bachelor's degree in advanced courses in health, math, and science. As part of their graduate curriculum, optometrists concentrate specifically on the structure, function, and disorders of the eye. They also study general health, anatomy, physiology, and biochemistry, so they have an understanding of how a patient's overall medical condition can relate to eye health. Some optometrists specialize in geriatrics (care of older persons). An optometrist must be licensed by the state to practice and must earn continuing education credits to be able to renew licensure.

An optometrist conducts comprehensive eye exams, including screening for glaucoma, cataracts, and retinal diseases like macular degeneration and diabetic retinopathy. When an optometrist identifies any of these concerns, he or she will refer the patient to an ophthalmologist (see below) for specific treatment and care. An optometrist also prescribes corrective lenses and can fit people with eyeglasses or contact lenses.

An *ophthalmologist* is a medical doctor who specializes in health of the eye. Ophthalmologists are trained to provide the full spectrum of eye care, from prescribing eyeglasses and contact lenses to diagnosing eye diseases and performing complex and delicate eye surgery. They may also be engaged in scientific research.

An *optician* is a professional who makes eyeglass lenses from a prescription supplied by a doctor of optometry or an ophthalmologist.

When you get new corrective lenses, it may take some time to adjust to them. As indicated in Chapter 2, new vision correction can sometimes become a risk factor for falls. If you don't adjust within a few days to a week, let the doctor know. There could be an error in the prescription, in the positioning of the lens in relation to your eye, or in how the lenses were made.

DON'T FORGET YOUR FEET

In Chapter 2, on falls, I stressed the importance of keeping your feet in good condition and explained how feet can affect balance and gait. Another kind of doctor you might see is a *podiatrist*. Podiatrists are medical doctors who specialize in care of the feet, ankles, and lower legs. Podiatrists must have a medical degree (DPM, doctor of podiatric medicine) and must be licensed to practice. Often podiatrists are consulted for routine care only when a patient has a disease, like diabetes, that affects peripheral sensation. But many older people have trouble taking good care of their feet for a variety of reasons, including one as simple as no longer being able to reach their feet. If this is true for you and your feet are otherwise healthy, consider having your toenails cared for at a reputable salon or spa that gives pedicures. However, if you have any systemic disease, like diabetes, or have sores on your feet or legs, or if you are concerned about your feet for any reason, consult a podiatrist first.

LAST BUT NOT LEAST, DON'T FORGET YOUR TEETH

In 2004, Kavita Ahluwalia, D.D.S., M.P.H., of the School of Dental and Oral Surgery at Columbia University in New York, wrote in a professional publication about her concern for oral care among aging Americans. She expressed her feeling that we had failed, as a society, to provide quality and accessible dental care for our older population. In the pre-fluoride era, she noted, adults routinely lost all or most of their teeth by midlife. Although today most seniors have retained most of their teeth, they are at increased risk for periodontal diseases, which are associated with chronic diseases such as cardiovascular disease, cerebrovascular diseases, and diabetes. Given that the number and proportion of seniors in the population is increasing, the situation is likely to get worse over the next several decades.

Good oral care not only improves the condition of the mouth but also improves overall health and well-being. We have already discussed the role of teeth in eating, chewing, and choking prevention (see Chapter 5), but, as Dr. Ahluwalia points out, oral diseases and dysfunction can also affect speaking and social interactions. Based on what we know of the importance of social interactions to overall health, the consequences of bad oral care could also include increased isolation and depression.

Dr. Ahluwalia recommended these steps to address the situation.

> First, the financing and provision of oral health care must be integrated with the mechanisms used to ensure overall health and well-being for the elderly. Second, because seniors are more likely to visit a physician than a dentist, it is imperative that primary care providers and geriatricians be educated about the medical, functional, emotional, and social consequences of oral diseases and dysfunction and that they provide regular screening and preventive education for dental diseases. Third, the daily caretakers of homebound and institutionalized elderly—nurses, home care workers, and nurses' aides—need improved oral health care education and training. Fourth, quality assurance measures used by organizations that provide care for seniors ought to address oral health and function.

Finally, she noted that the dental community must recognize that managing oral diseases in older people poses specific challenges, which means that we must create new options for delivering improved oral health care to older people.

Most of these suggestions are aimed at health care policy makers, but there are personal policies we can follow as individuals to take care of our teeth. Visit your dentist, every six months, ideally. When in doubt, ask for instruction in proper brushing and flossing technique and frequency. Dental hygienists gladly give such guidance; they know how beneficial good dental habits are.

Whenever you see any type of doctor, try to think about your health as whole mind–whole body health. The more doctors know about your lifestyle, illnesses, medications, and dietary and exercise regimens, the better they will be able to diagnose your problems and treat you. And the healthier you are, the safer you will be.

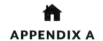

INJURY STATISTICS
FOR PEOPLE 65 AND OLDER

The U.S. Consumer Product Safety Commission (CPSC) collects injury data associated with about 15,000 consumer products. Below is a table of product categories for which 25 percent or more of the associated injuries happened to people 65 or older. The table shows the total estimated number of injuries (all ages) associated with each product category and the estimated number to those 65 and older. The list is arranged in order of decreasing number of injuries to that older population. The data are from 2010. Common injury scenarios among the 65 and older population are noted.

This table was created using data from CPSC's NEISS system. NEISS (National Electronic Injury Surveillance System) is a database of consumer product–related injuries reported to CPSC from approximately 100 hospital emergency departments throughout the United States. These hospitals constitute a statistically valid sample from which the CPSC estimates the number of product-related injuries on a national level. For the purposes of this book, I have omitted details on the statistical error expected with these figures, but readers are asked to bear in mind that the actual number of injuries could be somewhat smaller or larger than the estimated number shown.

Table A.1. Injuries Reported in 2010

Product code*	Product category	Estimated total injuries	Estimated injuries to 65+	Primary injury scenario for 65+
1807	Floors	1,366,423	542,470	Fell to the floor
4076	Beds or bed frames	639,303	212,249	Rolled out of bed, or fell getting out of bed
4074	Chairs, not specified	354,994	113,598	Fell out of chair
1706	Crutches, canes, walkers	133,527	102,949	Fell while using, or tripped over and fell
1707	Wheelchairs	145,850	96,699	Fell out of
0649	Toilets	103,998	53,767	Fell off of or fell onto
0676	Rugs or carpets, unspecified	120,873	49,921	Tripped on, including tripped while using walker
1878	Door frames or sills	60,620	16,125	Fell, striking door frame
1645	Daywear	61,276	16,054	Fell getting dressed or undressed
0841	Bench or table saws	32,669	10,846	Laceration or amputation of thumb, fingers
1212	Golf activity, apparel or equipment	35,199	10,243	Developed chest pain while playing
0612	Throw rugs, runners, doormats	19,490	9,998	Tripped on and fell
0670	Recliner chairs	23,961	9,656	Fell getting out of, or slipped out of
0648	Sinks	31,699	8,305	Fell and struck

Table A.1. *Continued*

Product code*	Product category	Estimated total injuries	Estimated injuries to 65+	Primary injury scenario for 65+
4080	Stools	27,832	8,099	Fell off; fell when wheeled stool slipped as person tried to sit on it
0550	Telephones or telephone accessories	20,885	7,205	Tripped over cord; or got up to answer phone, lost balance, and fell
1606	Eyeglasses	16,735	6,778	When person fell, eyeglasses cut into face, especially bridge of nose
0620	Step stools	14,660	6,055	Fell off of
1414	Garden hoses, nozzles, sprinklers	14,942	5,514	Tripped over hose or sprinkler
1744	Motorized vehicles, 3+ wheels (mobility devices and scooters used, for example, in stores and homes)	9,175	5,340	Crash, steering mishap
1623	Luggage	17,041	5,027	Strain from lifting, or fell over piece of
1843	Ramps or landings	16,162	4,913	Slipped, tripped, or fell on
0613	Wall-to-wall carpeting	13,946	4,770	Fell onto
0618	Step ladders	11,671	4,213	Fell off of
4081	Electrical cords	10,083	4,033	Tripped over and fell
1890	Escalators	12,463	3,926	Tripped, fell, or lost balance on

Continued

Table A.1. *Continued*

Product code*	Product category	Estimated total injuries	Estimated injuries to 65+	Primary injury scenario for 65+
1889	Elevators	11,201	3,114	Door closed on person or person tripped getting into or out of elevator; knocked person down
1465	Decorative yard equipment	11,620	3,033	Fell onto mailbox
0214	Dishwashers	9,239	2,652	Tripped over open door and fell
4079	Footstools, ottomans, hassocks	8,768	2,499	Tripped over or fell off of
4051	Sheets or pillow cases	6,619	2,469	Got tangled in or tripped over
0689	Blankets, unspecified	7,721	2,455	Tripped on and fell
1620	Hearing aids	3,447	2,099	Part of hearing aid stuck in ear
1644	Nightwear	5,452	1,995	Tripped on pajamas, robe, nightgown; fell while putting on pajamas
0617	Draperies, curtains, shower curtains	6,679	1,690	Fell off chair, stool, or bed while hanging curtain
4068	Scales	2,375	1,309	Lost balance getting on or off scale and fell
4008	Nonelectric blankets	3,523	1,166	Got tangled in or tripped over
0638	Window blinds or shades	3,766	1,103	Laceration while cleaning

Table A.1. *Continued*

Product code*	Product category	Estimated total injuries	Estimated injuries to 65+	Primary injury scenario for 65+
0110	Electric heating pads	4,006	1,078	Burns associated with falling asleep on the pad
0667	Bedspreads or throws	2,219	834	Tripped over or got tangled in and fell
4042	Lighting equipment, not specified	3,036	829	Reaching to turn off lights, lost balance, fell
1808	Outdoor awnings, shutters	2,530	827	Various, associated with installing or adjusting awnings
0112	Sewing machines	2,698	796	Dropped or fell into the machine
1821	Clothesline or clothes drying rack	2,452	689	Fell while taking clothes off line; fell into clothes rack
0137	Automatic doors	1,759	536	Door closed on person or knocked person down
0434	Doorstops	1,300	536	Tripped over doorstop or fell onto it
1405	Garden tractors	1,814	517	Vehicle rolled over on hill; person lost balance and fell from
1136	Canning jars or lids	1,656	502	Fell carrying jars; person overheated
0854	Workshop furnishings	1,877	471	Various, mostly involving a workbench
0408	Ironing boards or covers	1,578	426	Tripped and fell into board

Continued

Table A.1. *Continued*

Product code*	Product category	Estimated total injuries	Estimated injuries to 65+	Primary injury scenario for 65+
1455	Manual pruning or trimming equipment, not specified	1,414	396	Laceration, or fell from ladder or stool while trimming bushes
1453	Other manual pruning or trimming equipment	1,521	395	Cut while trimming bushes
1449	Manual hedge trimmers	1,355	371	Cut while trimming bushes
0231	Electric mixers	1,262	366	Hand caught in beaters or injured when mixer dropped onto self

*The NEISS Product Code, assigned by the CPSC

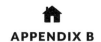

APPENDIX B

AGENCIES AND ORGANIZATIONS THAT CAN HELP

There are many, many sources of information on aging well and staying safe—too many to cite in a single list. While this appendix is not comprehensive, it lists key government agencies and other organizations that offer up-to-date information and recommendations. The list is organized alphabetically by category and provides a brief description of the resource. Some agencies and organizations are included under more than one category. If you search on your own, you will most certainly find many more sources of good information.

AGING IN GENERAL

AARP (formerly the American Association of Retired Persons)
601 E Street, NW, Washington, DC 20049
888-OUR-AARP (888-687-2277)
www.aarp.org

AARP is a nonprofit, nonpartisan membership organization for people ages 50 and over. The organization is dedicated to enhancing quality of life for all Americans as they age. It campaigns for what it views as positive social changes and delivers value to members through information, advocacy, and service.

Administration on Aging
c/o Administration on Community Living
1 Massachusetts Avenue, NW, Washington, DC 20001
Public inquiries: 202-619-0724
Eldercare locator (to find local resources): 800-677-1116
www.aoa.gov

The mission of the Administration on Aging is to develop a comprehensive, coordinated, and cost-effective system of home and community-based services that helps elderly individuals maintain their health and independence in their homes and communities.

The American Geriatrics Society (AGS)
The Empire State Building
350 Fifth Avenue, Suite 801, New York, NY 10118-0801
212-308-1414
http://americangeriatrics.org/public_education/

The AGS Foundation for Health in Aging was established by the American Geriatrics Society in 1999 to bring the expertise of geriatrics and gerontological health professionals to the public. The foundation draws on the expertise of AGS members to provide comprehensive information on the common diseases and disorders of older adults. The AGS Foundation for Health in Aging's flagship initiative is the Health in Aging website, a one-stop, comprehensive source of up-to-date information about what to do to stay healthy and what to do when health problems arise in later life.

Exercise and Physical Activity: Your Everyday Guide
from the National Institute on Aging
www.nia.nih.gov/health/publication/exercise-physical-activity
-your-everyday-guide-national-institute-aging-1

This 120-page guide describes the benefits of exercise and physical activity for older people. Learn how to set exercise goals and stick to them. Includes samples of exercises for endurance, strength, balance, and flexibility and a list of other resources.

National Institute on Aging
31 Center Drive, MSC 2292, Bethesda, MD 20892
800-222-2225 (TTY, 800-222-4225)
www.nia.nih.gov

The institute provides general information on research and practical resources for the aging population. To sign up for regular e-mail alerts about new publications and other information, go to www.nia.nih.gov/HealthInformation. (See also next entry.)

National Institute on Aging Information Center
P.O. Box 8057, Gaithersburg, MD 20898-8057
800-222-2225 (TTY, 800-222-4225)
www.nihseniorhealth.gov

The National Institutes of Health's Senior Health website makes aging-related health information easily accessible for people seeking reliable, easy-to-understand, online health information. Special features make it simple to use. For example, you can click on a button to have the text read out loud or to make the type larger. This site was developed by the National Institute on Aging and the National Library of Medicine, both parts of the National Institutes of Health (NIH).

ALZHEIMER'S DISEASE

Alzheimer's Association
225 North Michigan Avenue, Suite 1700, Chicago, IL 60601-7633
800-272-3900
www.alz.org

The Alzheimer's Association is the leading, global health organization giving support to caregivers and families of people with Alzheimer's disease, and it is the largest private, nonprofit funder of Alzheimer's disease research.

Alzheimer's Disease Education and Referral (ADEAR) Center
National Institute on Aging, P.O. Box 8250,
Silver Spring, MD 20907-8250
800-438-4380
www.nia.nih.gov/Alzheimers

The National Institute on Aging leads the federal government in conducting and supporting research on aging and the health and well-being of older people. The referenced segment of the website is devoted to Alzheimer's disease. The ADEAR Center offers information and publications for families, caregivers, and professionals on diagnosis, treatment, patient care, caregiver needs, long-term care, education and training, and research related to Alzheimer's disease.

Home Safety for People with Alzheimer's Disease
Dec. 2008; NIH Publication #02-5179 NIA
www.nia.nih.gov/sites/default/files/home_safety_for_people_with
_alzheimers_disease.pdf

This is a 44-page booklet from the National Institute on Aging.

Medic Alert Foundation + Safe Return
2323 Colorado Avenue, Turlock, CA 95282
888-633-4298
www.medicalert.org.

This is a 24-hour, nationwide emergency response service for individuals with Alzheimer's or a related dementia who wander or have a medical emergency. Members of this program are identified by a piece of jewelry, like a bracelet or necklace, that they wear that provides an emergency phone number to call. The response center can identify the member's contacts, making sure the person is returned home.

CAREGIVER SUPPORT

Children of Aging Parents
P.O. Box 167, Richboro, PA 18954
800-227-7294
www.caps4caregivers.org

This nonprofit group provides information and materials for adult children caring for elderly parents. Other caregivers may also find this information helpful.

ElderCare Online
50 Amuxen Court, Islip, NY 11751
www.ec-online.net

This website features information, education, and support for caregivers, including safety advice, and links to additional caregiver resources. It is maintained by Prism Innovations, Inc., publishers of information for people ages 50 and older.

Eldercare Locator
800-677-1116
www.eldercare.gov

Eldercare Locator is a nationwide directory-assistance service helping older people and their caregivers locate local support and resources. It is funded by the Administration on Aging, whose website
at www.aoa.gov also features Alzheimer's disease information for
families, caregivers, and health professionals.

Family Caregiver Alliance
180 Montgomery Street, Suite 1100, San Francisco, CA 94104
800-445-8106
www.caregiver.org

The Family Caregiver Alliance is a nonprofit organization that offers
support services and information for people caring for people with
Alzheimer's, stroke, traumatic brain injuries, and other cognitive
disorders.

Well Spouse Association
63 West Main Street, Suite H, Freehold, NJ 07728
800-838-0879
www.wellspouse.org

This nonprofit organization gives support to spouses and partners
of people who are chronically ill and/or disabled. Among its offer-
ings are support groups and a newsletter.

DRIVING

AAA Foundation for Traffic Safety, Administrative Office
607 14th Street, NW, Suite 201, Washington, DC 20005-2000
202-638-5944
www.seniordrivers.org

This nonprofit foundation dedicated to traffic safety research and
education maintains a website that provides information and tools
to help seniors drive safely longer. It helps seniors evaluate and improve their driving skills and offers resources for family and friends.

American Association of Motor Vehicle Administrators
4301 Wilson Boulevard, Suite 400, Arlington, VA 22203
703-522-4200
www.granddriver.info

GrandDriver is a pilot program that provides information about aging and driving. It focuses on drivers over 65 and their adult children, urging both groups to learn more about the effects of aging on our ability to drive and to talk about these issues.

Centers for Disease Control and Prevention,
National Center for Injury Prevention
4770 Buford Highway, NE, Atlanta, GA 30341-3717
800-232-4636
www.cdc.gov/motorvehiclesafety/Older_Adult_Drivers/index.html

This website provides up-to-date data and statistics on older drivers.

DriveWise
Beth Israel Deaconess Medical Center
330 Brookline Avenue, Boston, MA 02215
617-667-4074
Main Switchboard: 617-667-7000
Find a Doctor: 800-667-5356
Directions by Phone: 617-667-3000
TDD (for hearing impaired): 800-439-0183
www.bidmc.org/CentersandDepartments/Departments/Neurology
/CognitiveNeurology/Drivewise.aspx

The goal of the DriveWise program at Beth Israel Deaconess Medical Center is to provide objective information about driving safety while providing support for individuals and their families.

Driving Decisions Workbook
by D. W. Eby, University of Michigan Ann Arbor, Transportation Research Institute, Social and Behavioral Analysis Division, 2000
http://hdl.handle.net/2027.42/1321;
www.umtri.umich.edu/library/pdf/2000-14.pdf

An interactive tool to help you evaluate and improve driving skills.

Federal Highway Administration
Office of Safety–HSST
1200 New Jersey Avenue, SE, Washington, DC 20590
202-366-6836
http://safety.fhwa.dot.gov/older_users/

At this web address, the FHA has information on an older driver's program.

The Hartford
Hartford Plaza
690 Asylum Avenue, Hartford, CT 06115
860-547-5000
www.thehartford.com/alzheimers

This website offering Alzheimer's information, in the section "Dementia and Driving," helps drivers with dementia and their families plan a successful transition from driver to passenger.

FEDERAL GOVERNMENT AGENCIES AND RESOURCES

Administration on Aging
c/o Administration on Community Living
1 Massachusetts Avenue, NW, Washington, DC 20001
Public inquiries: 202-619-0724
Eldercare locator (to find local resources): (800) 677-1116
www.aoa.gov

The mission of the Administration on Aging is to develop a comprehensive, coordinated, and cost-effective system of home and community-based services that helps elderly individuals maintain their health and independence in their homes and communities.

Centers for Medicare and Medicaid Services
7500 Security Boulevard, Baltimore, MD 21244-1850
800-MEDICARE (800-633-4227) (TTY/TDD, 877-486-2048)
www.medicare.gov

Food and Drug Administration (FDA)
10903 New Hampshire Avenue, Silver Spring, MD 20993-0002
888-463-6332, 888-INFO-FDA
www.fda.gov

MedlinePlus
c/o National Library of Medicine
8600 Rockville Pike, Bethesda, MD 20894
888-FIND-NLM (888-346-3656)
www.medlineplus.gov

MedlinePlus is the National Institutes of Health's medical information website for nonprofessionals. Produced by the National Library
of Medicine, it provides information about diseases, medical conditions, and wellness issues in language laypeople can understand.
MedlinePlus offers reliable, up-to-date health information.

MedlinePlus provides access to extensive information from the
National Institutes of Health and other trusted sources on more
than 900 diseases and conditions. There are directories; a medical encyclopedia and a medical dictionary; easy-to-understand
tutorials on common conditions, tests, and treatments; health information in Spanish; extensive information on prescription and
nonprescription drugs; health information from the media; and
links to thousands of clinical trials. MedlinePlus is updated daily.
There is no advertising on this site, nor does MedlinePlus endorse
any company or product.

National Eye Institute
31 Center Drive, Bethesda, MD 20892-2510
301-496-5248
www.nei.nih.gov

National Institute on Aging
31 Center Drive, MSC 2292, Bethesda, MD 20892
800-222-2225 (TTY, 800-222-4225)
www.nia.nih.gov

The Institute on Aging provides general information on research
and practical resources for the aging population. To sign up for

regular e-mail alerts about new publications and other information, go to www.nia.nih.gov/HealthInformation. (See also next entry.)

National Institute on Aging Information Center
P.O. Box 8057, Gaithersburg, MD 20898-8057
1-800-222-2225 (TTY, 800-222-4225)
www.nihseniorhealth.gov

This website offers health and wellness information for older adults. It makes aging-related health information easily accessible for people seeking reliable, easy-to-understand, online health information. This site was developed by the National Institute on Aging and the National Library of Medicine, both part of the National Institutes of Health.

National Institute on Deafness and
Other Communication Disorders
Information Clearinghouse
1 Communication Avenue, Bethesda, MD 20892-3456
800-241-1044 (TTY, 800-241-1055)
www.nidcd.nih.gov

U.S. Consumer Product Safety Commission
4330 East West Highway, Bethesda, MD 20814
Consumer Hotline: 800-638-2772 (TTY, 301-595-7054)
www.cpsc.gov

FIRE AND ELECTRICAL SAFETY

Electrical Safety Foundation International
1300 North 17th Street, Suite 1752, Rosslyn, VA 22209
703-841-3229
http://esfi.org

The Electrical Safety Foundation International is the premier nonprofit organization dedicated exclusively to promoting electrical safety at home and in the workplace.

National Fire Protection Association (NFPA)
1 Batterymarch Park, Quincy, MA 02169-7471
617-770-3000
www.nfpa.org

Established in 1896, the NFPA is the world's leading advocate of fire prevention and an authoritative source on public safety. NFPA develops, publishes, and disseminates more than 300 consensus codes and standards intended to minimize the possibility and effects of fire and other risks.

FOOD SAFETY

Choking information: nsc.org/SAFETY_HOME/HOMEAND RECREATIONALSAFETY/Pages/Choking.aspx

Common sources of food poisoning: foodsafety.gov/poisoning /index.html

Egg storage information: foodsafety.gov/keep/charts /eggstorage.html

Food and power outages: bt.cdc.gov/disasters/poweroutage /needtoknow.asp

Food safety for the elderly: fsis.usda.gov/PDF/Food_Safety_for _Older_Adults.pdf

Food storage times in the fridge: foodsafety.gov/keep/charts /storagetimes.html

General safe food handling and preparing: fightbac.org/safe-food -handling; foodsafety.gov/keep/types/index.html; and foodsafety .gov/keep/preparing/index.html

Poisoning in the United States: Fact Sheet: cdc.gov/homeand recreationalsafety/poisoning/poisoning-factsheet.htm

Unintentional poisoning: Centers for Disease Control and Prevention. cdc.gov/HomeandRecreationalSafety/Poisoning/index.html

HEARING AND SPEECH

American Academy of Audiology
11730 Plaza America Drive, Suite 300, Reston, VA 20190
800-AAA-2336
www.audiology.org

American Speech-Language-Hearing Association
2200 Research Boulevard, Rockville, MD 20850-3289
800-638-8255 (TTY, 301-296-5650)
www.asha.org/public/

The American Speech-Language-Hearing Association is committed to ensuring that all people with speech, language, and hearing disorders receive services to help them communicate effectively. The referenced segment of the website for the general public provides resources to help you understand communication and communication disorders.

American Tinnitus Association
522 SW Fifth Avenue, Suite 825, Portland, OR 97204
Mailing address: P.O. Box 5, Portland, OR 97207-0005
800-634-8978
www.ata.org

This association provides current information on tinnitus. Its mission is to cure tinnitus through the development of resources that advance tinnitus research.

Federal Trade Commission advice on hearing aids: ftc.gov/bcp/edu
/pubs/consumer/health/hea10.shtm and ftc.gov/whocares

Food and Drug Administration information on hearing aids:
fda.gov/MedicalDevices/ProductsandMedicalProcedures/Home
HealthandConsumer/ConsumerProducts/HearingAids/default.htm

Hearing Loop

www.HearingLoop.org

Hearing Loop is a nonprofit informational website created and maintained by Hope College. "Get in the Hearing Loop" is a campaign endorsed by the American Academy of Audiology and the Hearing Loss Association of America to educate and excite hearing aid users, as well as audiologists and other professionals who dispense hearing aids, about telecoils and hearing loops and their unique benefits.

Hearing Loss Association of America

7910 Woodmont Avenue, Suite 1200, Bethesda, MD 20814

301-657-2248 (TTY, 301-657-2249)

www.hearingloss.org

The Hearing Loss Association of America (HLAA) is the nation's leading organization representing people with hearing loss. HLAA provides assistance and resources for people with hearing loss and their families to learn how to adjust to living with hearing loss. HLAA is working to eradicate the stigma associated with hearing loss and raise public awareness about the need for prevention, treatment, and regular hearing screenings throughout life.

"How's Your Hearing?"

www.HowsYourHearing.org

"How's Your Hearing?" is a consumer-friendly website developed by the American Academy of Audiology to give consumers an overview of hearing, hearing loss, hearing aids, common conditions, and more. The site has a "Find an Audiologist" directory to help you locate an audiologist near you.

**National Institute on Deafness and
Other Communication Disorders
Information Clearinghouse**
1 Communication Avenue, Bethesda, MD 20892-3456
800-241-1044 (TTY, 800-241-1055)
www.nidcd.nih.gov

Telecoil information: nchearingloss.org/telecoil.htm?fromncshhh

VISION

National Eye Institute
31 Center Drive, Bethesda, MD 20892-2510
www.nei.nih.gov/health/

This website provides eye health information for the general public.

REFERENCES

Chapter 1. What's "Old" Got to Do with It?

Bergen G, Chen LH, Warner M, Fingerhut LA. *Injury in the United States: 2007 Chartbook*. Hyattsville, MD: National Center for Health Statistics; 2008.

Bonfils P, Faulcon P, Tavernier L, et al. Home accidents associated with anosmia. *Presse Med*. 2008;37(5 Pt 1):742–45. ePub; DOI: 10.1016/j.lpm .2007.09.028.

The changing brain in healthy aging. nia.nih.gov/alzheimers/publication /part-1-basics-healthy-brain/changing-brain-healthy-aging.

Development, growth, and senescence in the chemical senses. US Department of Health and Human Services, conference proceedings. NIH publication 93-3483. Bethesda, MD: National Institutes of Health; 1992.

Glisky EL. Changes in cognitive function in human aging. In *Frontiers in Neuroscience*. Boca Raton, FL: CRC Press, Taylor & Francis Group; 2007.

Home safety for people with Alzheimer's disease. NIH Publication 02-5179. Bethesda, MD: National Institute on Aging; Dec. 2008.

Horan MA, Little RA, eds. *Injury in the Aging*. Cambridge: Cambridge University Press; 1998.

National Center for Injury Prevention and Control. *Injury Fact Book, 2001–2002*. Atlanta, GA: Centers for Disease Control and Prevention; 2001.

Nayak USL. How can products be made safer for use by older people? *Int J Consumer & Product Safety*. 1998;5(2):91–98.

Plassman BL, Langa KM, Fisher GG, Heeringa SG, Weir DR, Ofstedal MB, Burke JR, Hurd MD, et al. Prevalence of dementia in the United States: the aging, demographics, and memory study. *Neuroepidemiology*. 2007;29(1–2):125–32.

Rutherford GW Jr., Marcy N, Mills A. *Hazard Screening Report: Injuries to Persons 65 Years of Age and Older*. Washington, DC: US Consumer Product Safety Commission; Oct. 2004.

Sleet DA, Ballesteros MF, Baldwin GT. Injuries: an under-recognized lifestyle problem. *Amer J Lifestyle Med*. 2010;4:8–15. DOI: 10.1177/155982760 9348343.

Smith TP. Older consumer safety: phase I. Project report, US Consumer Product Safety Commission, Division of Human Factors. Washington, DC: USCPSC; 2005.

Swanson J, ed. *Physical and Mental Issues in Aging Sourcebook*. Detroit, MI: Omnigraphics; 1999.

Turner S, Arthur G, Lyons RA, Weightman AL, Mann MK, Jones SJ, John A, Lannon S. Modification of the home environment for the reduction of injuries. Review. *Cochrane Database Syst Rev*. 2011;Feb. 16;(2):CD003600.

US Consumer Product Safety Commission. Emergency room treated injuries: adults 65 and over. Special report. Washington, DC: USCPSC; 2004.

Vidal S, Werner CA. The older population 2010. US Census. Census Bureau webinar, Nov. 30, 2011.

Wan H, Sengupta M, Velkoff V, DeBarros K. *US Census Bureau, Current Population Reports, P23-209, 65+ in the United States: 2005*. Washington, DC: US Government Printing Office; 2005.

Chapter 2. Don't Fall!

Atay E, Akeniz M. Falls in elderly: fear of falling and physical activity. *GeroFam* 2011;2(1):11–28.

Beauchet O, Annweiler C, Verghese J, Fantino B, Herrmann FR, Allali G. Biology of gait control: vitamin D involvement. *Neurology*. 2011;May 10;76(19):1617–22.

Bergen G, Chen LH, Warner M, Fingerhut LA. *Injury in the United States: 2007 Chartbook*. Hyattsville, MD: National Center for Health Statistics; 2008.

Berlie HD, Garwood CL. Diabetes medications related to an increased risk of falls and fall-related morbidity in the elderly. *Ann Pharmacother*. 2010;Apr.;44(4):712–17.

Blalock SJ, Demby KB, McCulloch KL, Stevens JA. Factors influencing hip protector use among community-dwelling older adults. *Injury Prevention*. 2010;16:235–39.

Boyd R, Stevens J. Falls and fear of falling: burden, beliefs and behaviours. *Age Ageing*. 2009;Jul.;38(4):423–28.

Bradley SM. Falls in older adults. *Mt. Sinai J Med*. 2011;78(4):590–95.

Butler AA, Lord SR, Fitzpatrick RC. Reach distance but not judgment error is associated with falls in older people. *J Gerontol A Biol Sci Med Sci*. 2011;Aug.;66(8):896–903.

Carpenter CR, Scheatzle MD, D'Antonio JA, Ricci PT, Coben JH. Identification of fall risk factors in older adult emergency department patients. *Acad Emerg Med*. 2009;16(3):211–19.

Cashin RP, Yang M. Medications prescribed and occurrence of falls in general medicine inpatients. *Can J Hosp Pharm*. 2011;64(5):321–26.

Centers for Disease Control and Prevention. Nonfatal fall-related injuries associated with dogs and cats—United States, 2001–2006. *MMWR Morb Mortal Wkly Rep*. 2009;Mar. 27;58(11):277–81.

Centers for Disease Control and Prevention. Reasons for not seeking eye care among adults aged ≥40 years with moderate-to-severe visual impairment—21 States, 2006–2009. *MMWR Morb Mortal Wkly Rep.* 2011; 60(19):610–13.

Chapman GJ, Scally AJ, Elliott DB. Adaptive gait changes in older people due to lens magnification. *Ophthalmic Physiol Opt.* 2011;31(3):311–17.

Chiarelli PE, Mackenzie LA, Osmotherly PG. Urinary incontinence is associated with an increase in falls: a systematic review. *Aust J Physiother.* 2009;55(2):89–95.

Dickinson A, Machen I, Horton K, Jain D, Maddex T, Cove J. Fall prevention in the community: what older people say they need. *Br J Community Nurs.* 2011;16(4):174–80.

Dindyal S, Bhuva N, Kumaraswamy P, Khoshnaw H. Falls in the elderly—the need for more access to chiropody. Letter. *Age and Ageing.* 2009;38: 127–28. DOI: 10.1093/ageing/afn243.

Downton JH. Who falls and why? In *Injury in the Aging.* Edited by MA Horan and RA Little. Cambridge: Cambridge University Press; 1998.

Faulkner KA, Cauley JA, Studenski SA, Landsittel DP, Cummings SR, Ensrud KE, Donaldson MG, Nevitt MC (Study of Osteoporotic Fractures Research Group). Lifestyle predicts falls independent of physical risk factors. *Osteoporos Int.* 2009;Dec.;20(12):2025–34.

Filiatrault J, Desrosiers J. Coping strategies used by seniors going through the normal aging process: does fear of falling matter? *Gerontology.* 2011;57(3):228–36.

Gillespie L, Handoll H. Prevention of falls and fall-related injuries in older people. *Injury Prevention.* 2009;15(5):354–55.

Gribbin J, Hubbard R, Gladman J, Smith C, Lewis S. Risk of falls associated with antihypertensive medication: self-controlled case series. *Pharmacoepidemiol Drug Saf.* 2011;Aug.;20(8):879–84.

Hegeman J, van den Bemt BJ, Duysens J, van Limbeek J. NSAIDs and the risk of accidental falls in the elderly: a systematic review. *J Drug Safety.* 2009;32(6):489–98.

Intlekofer K. Stop that. *Johns Hopkins University Alumni Magazine.* Winter 2011:50–57.

Källstrand-Ericson J, Hildingh C. Visual impairment and falls: a register study. *J Clin Nurs.* 2009;18(3):366–72.

Kojima T, Akishita M, Nakamura T, Nomura K, Ogawa S, Iijima K, Eto M, Ouchi Y. Association of polypharmacy with fall risk among geriatric outpatients. *Geriatr Gerontol Int.* 2011;11(4):438–44.

Kurrle SE, Day R, Cameron ID. The perils of pet ownership: a new fall-injury risk factor. *Med J Aust.* 2004;Dec.6–20;181(11–12):682–83.

Laing SS, Silver IF, York S, Phelan EA. Fall prevention knowledge, attitude, and practices of community stakeholders and older adults. *J Aging Research Epub.* 2011; Sep. 7; article ID 395357, 9 pages. DOI:10.4061/2011/ 395357.

Lamoth CJ, Caljouw SR, Postema K. Active video gaming to improve balance in the elderly. *Stud Health Technol Inform*. 2011;167:159–64.

Lamoureux E, Gadgil S, Pesudovs K, Keeffe J, Fenwick E, Salonen S, Rees G, Dirani M. The relationship between visual function, duration and main causes of vision loss and falls in older people with low vision. *Graefes Arch Clin Exp Ophthalmol*. 2010;Apr.;248(4):527–33.

Legood R, Scuffham C, Cryer C. Are we blind to injuries in the visually impaired? A review of the literature. *Injury Prevention*. 2002;8:155–60.

Lin FR, Ferrucci L. Hearing loss and falls among older adults in the United States. *Arch Intern Med*. 2012;172(4):369–71. DOI:10.1001/archinternmed. 2011.728.

Liu-Ambrose T, Nagamatsu LS, Hsu CL, Bolandzadeh N. Emerging concept: 'central benefit model' of exercise in falls prevention. *Br J Sports Med*. 2012; Apr. 20; ePub.

Mahler M, Sarvimäki A. Fear of falling from a daily life perspective: narratives from later life. *Scand J Caring Sc*. 2012;Mar.;26(1):38–44.

Menz HB, Hill KD. Podiatric involvement in multidisciplinary falls-prevention clinics in Australia. *J Am Podiatr Med Assoc*. 2007;Sep.–Oct.; 97(5):377–84.

Modreker MK, von Renteln-Kruse W. Medication and falls in old age. *Internist*. 2009;Apr.;50(4):493–500.

Moncada LV. Management of falls in older persons: a prescription for prevention. *Am Fam Physician*. 2011;84(11):267–76.

Narayanan MR, Scalzi ME, Redmond SJ, Lord SR, Celler BG, Lovell NH. Evaluation of functional deficits and falls risk in the elderly—methods for preventing falls. *Conf Proc IEEE Eng Med Biol Soc*. 2009;1:6179–82.

National Institute on Aging. Safety for people with Alzheimer's disease. NIH publication number 02-5179. Bethesda, MD: National Institute on Aging; Dec. 2008.

Panel on Prevention of Falls in Older Persons, American Geriatrics Society and British Geriatrics Society. Summary of the updated American Geriatrics Society/British Geriatrics Society clinical practice guideline for prevention of falls in older persons. *J Amer Geriatrics Soc*. 2011;Jan.; 59(1):148–57. onlinelibrary.wiley.com/doi/10.1111/j.1532-5415.2010.03234 .x/full.

Planton J, Edlund BJ. Strategies for reducing polypharmacy in older adults. *J Gerontol Nurs*. 2010;Jan.;36(1):8–12. DOI: 10.3928/00989134-20091204-03.

Price JM. *Fall Injury Prevention for Older Adults—and Those Who Care about Them*. New York: iUniverse; 2007.

Pynoos J, Steinman BA, Nguyen AQ. Environmental assessment and modification as fall-prevention strategies for older adults. *Clin Geriatr Med*. 2010;26(4):633–44.

Rietdyk S, Rhea CK. The effect of the visual characteristics of obstacles on risk of tripping and gait parameters during locomotion. *Ophthalmic Physiol Opt*. 2011;31(3):302–10.

Roe B, Howell F, Riniotis K, Beech R, Crome P, Ong BN. Older people and falls: health status, quality of life, lifestyle, care networks, prevention and views on service use following a recent fall. *J Clin Nurs*. 2009;18(16): 2261–72.

Schulz BW, Lloyd JD, Lee WE. The effects of everyday concurrent tasks on overground minimum toe clearance and gait parameters. *Gait Posture*. 2010;May;32(1):18–22.

Secoli SR. Polypharmacy: interaction and adverse reactions in the use of drugs by elderly people. *Rev Bras Enferm*. 2010;63(1):136–40.

Shahar D, Levi M, Kurtz I, Shany S, Zvili I, Mualleme E, Shahar A, Sarid O, Melzer I. Nutritional status in relation to balance and falls in the elderly. A preliminary look at serum folate. *Ann Nutr Metab*. 2009;54(1):59–66.

Sherrington C, Whitney JC, Lord SR, Herbert RD, Cumming RG, Close JC. Effective exercise for the prevention of falls: a systematic review and meta-analysis. *J Am Geriatr Soc*. 2008;56(12):2234–43.

Smith TP. *Older Consumer Safety, Phase 1*. Washington, DC: US Consumer Product Safety Commission. Division of Human Factors. 2005.

Speechley M. Unintentional falls in older adults: a methodological historical review. *Can J Aging*. 2011;Mar.;1:1–12; ePub.

Spink MJ, Fotoohabadi MR, Wee E, Landorf KB, Hill KD, Lord SR, Menz HB. Predictors of adherence to a multifaceted podiatry intervention for the prevention of falls in older people. *BMC Geriatr*. 2011;11(1):51.

Stevens JA, Haas EN, Haileyesus T. Nonfatal bathroom injuries among persons aged ≥15years—United States, 2008. *J Saf Res*. 2011;42(4):311–15.

Stevens JA, Noonan RK, Rubenstein LZ. Older adult fall prevention: perceptions, beliefs, and behaviors. *Am J Lifestyle Med*. 2010;4(1):16–20.

Stevens JA, Thomas K, Teh L, Greenspan AI. Unintentional fall injuries associated with walkers and canes in older adults treated in U.S. emergency departments. *J Am Geriatr Soc*. 2009;Aug.;57(8):1464–69.

Swanson J, ed. *Physical and Mental Issues in Aging Sourcebook*, 1st ed. Detroit, MI: Omnigraphics; 1999.

Tinetti ME, Kumar C. The patient who falls: "It's always a trade-off." *JAMA*. 2010;303(3):258–66.

US Consumer Product Safety Commission. NEISS database, 2010. cpsc.gov /library/neiss.html.

Viswanathan A, Sudarsky L. Balance and gait problems in the elderly. *Handb Clin Neurol*. 2011;103:623–34.

Wan H, Sengupta M, Velkoff V, and DeBarros K. US Census Bureau, Current Population Reports, P23-209, 65+ in the United States: 2005. Washington, DC: US Government Printing Office; 2005.

Willmott H, Greenheld N, Goddard R. Beware of the dog? An observational study of dog-related musculoskeletal injury in the UK. *Accid Anal Prev.* 2012;May;46:52–54. Epub Jan. 25, 2012.

Wood J, Lacherez P, Black A, Cole M, Boon M, Kerr G. Risk of falls, injurious falls, and other injuries resulting from visual impairment among older adults with age-related macular degeneration. *Invest Ophthalmol Vis Sci.* 2011;Jul. 7;52(8):5088–92.

Chapter 3. Too Hot and Too Cold

Albornoz CR, Villegas J, Sylvester M, Peña V, Bravo I. Burns are more aggressive in the elderly: proportion of deep burn area / total burn area might have a role in mortality. *Burns.* 2011;Sep.;37(6):1058–61.

Allison SP. Thermoregulation, nutrition and injury in the elderly. In *Injury in the Aging.* Edited by MA Horan and RA Little. Cambridge: Cambridge University Press; 1998.

Bishai D, Lee S. Heightened risk of fire deaths among older African Americans and Native Americans. *Public Health Rep.* (1974) 2010;125(3): 406–13.

Bonfils P, Faulcon P, Tavernier L, Bonfils NA, Malinvaud D. Home accidents associated with anosmia. *Presse Med.* 2008;May;37(5, part 1):742–45.

Consumer and Corporate Affairs, Bureau of Consumer Affairs. Product safety and our aging society: design considerations for manufacturers and designers. Publication CCAC No. 10888 93-03. Canada, 1995.

Electrical Safety Foundation International. Know the dangers in your older home. (Booklet.) ESFI-know-the-dangers-in-your-older-home -booklet_english.pdf.

Firefighters guide to educating occupants on the hazards of smoking and home oxygen use. mass.gov/eopss/docs/dfs/osfm/pubed/flyers/ff-ed -guidelines.pdf.

Firepot information from US Consumer Product Safety Commission. cpsc.gov/BUSINFO/frnotices/fr12/firepot.pdf.

Hansen A, Bi P, Nitschke M, Pisaniello D, Newbury J, Kitson A. Older persons and heat-susceptibility: the role of health promotion in a changing climate. *Health Promot J Austr.* 2011;22(spec. no.):S17–20.

Hypothermia information. bt.cdc.gov/disasters/winter/staysafe/hypo thermia.asp.

Hypothermia information. emedicinehealth.com/hypothermia/article _em.htm.

Hypothermia information. mayoclinic.com/health/hypothermia/DS00333.

Hypothermia information. medicinenet.com/hypothermia/article.htm.

Hypothermia information. nlm.nih.gov/medlineplus/hypothermia.html.

Klein MB, Lezotte DC, Heltshe S, Fauerbach J, Holavanahalli RK, Rivara FP, Pham T, Engrav L. Functional and psychosocial outcomes of older adults after burn injury: results from a multicenter database of severe burn injury. *J Burn Care Res.* 2011;Jan.–Feb.;32(1):66–78.

Mack KA, Liller K. Home injuries: potential for prevention. *Am J Lifestyle Medicine.* 2010;4:75–81.

Murabit A, Tredget EE. Review of burn injuries secondary to home oxygen. *J Burn Care Res.* 2012;Mar.–Apr.;33(2):212-17.

National Fire Prevention Association/Centers for Disease Control and Prevention. Fire safety tips for older adults. nfpa.org/categoryList.asp ?categoryID=1419&URL=Safety%20Information/For%20consumers /Populations/Older%20adults.

Petition for glass-fronted fireplaces. cpsc.gov/LIBRARY/FOIA/FOIA11 /pubcom/gasfireplacecomml.pdf.

Thomas I, Bruck D. Awakening of sleeping people: a decade of research. *Fire Technol.* 2010;46(3):743–61.

US Consumer Product Safety Commission, AARP, National Association of State Fire Marshals. Fire safety checklist for older consumers.

US Consumer Product Safety Commission. New technology in gas water heaters can save lives: CPSC, GAMA say new heaters will prevent fires from flammable vapors. CPSC Press Release No. 03-158, July 8, 2003.

Watkins GM. Burns in the elderly. In *Injury in the Aging.* Edited by MA Horan and RA Little. Cambridge: Cambridge University Press; 1998.

Zanni GR. Thermal burns and scalds: clinical complications in the elderly. *Consult Pharm.* 2012;27(1):16–21.

Chapter 4. Poisoning

Bonfils P, Faulcon P, Tavernier L, Bonfils NA, Malinvaud D. Home accidents associated with anosmia. *Presse Med.* 2008;May;37(5, part 1):742–45.

Bronstein AC, Spyker DA, Cantilena LR Jr, Green JL, Rumack BH, Dart RC. 2010 annual report of the American Association of Poison Control Centers' National Poison Data System (NPDS): 28th annual report. *Clin Toxicol* (Phila). 2011;Dec.;49(10):910–41.

Centers for Disease Control and Prevention. Unintentional poisoning. cdc.gov/HomeandRecreationalSafety/Poisoning/index.html.

Common sources of food poisoning: foodsafety.gov/poisoning/index.html.

Egg storage information: foodsafety.gov/keep/charts/eggstorage.html.

Food safety during power outages: bt.cdc.gov/disasters/poweroutage /needtoknow.asp.

Food safety for the elderly: fsis.usda.gov/PDF/Food_Safety_for_Older _Adults.pdf.

Food storage times in the fridge: foodsafety.gov/keep/charts/storagetimes .html.

General safe food handling and preparing: fightbac.org/safe-food-handling; foodsafety.gov/keep/types/index.html; and foodsafety.gov/keep /preparing/index.html.

Gettings MA, Kiernan NE. Practices and perceptions of food safety among seniors who prepare meals at home. *J Nutr Educ*. 2001;May–Jun.;33(3): 148–54.

Hampson NB, Weaver LK. Residential carbon monoxide alarm use: opportunities for poisoning prevention. *J Environ. Health*. 2011;73(6):30–33.

Haselberger MB, Kroner BA. Drug poisoning in older patients: preventative and management strategies. *Drugs Aging*. 1995;Oct. 7;7(4):292–97.

Hayes BD, Klein-Schwartz W, Gonzales LF. Causes of therapeutic errors in older adults: evaluation of National Poison Center data. *J Am Geriatr Soc*. 2009;Apr.;57(4):653–58.

Hudson PK, Hartwell HJ. Food safety awareness of older people at home: a pilot study. *J R Soc Promot Health*. 2002;Sep.;122(3):165–69.

Kendall PA, Hillers VV, Medeiros LC. Food safety guidance for older adults. *Clin Infect Dis*. 2006;May 1;42(9):1298–304.

King ME, Damon SA. Attitudes about carbon monoxide safety in the United States: results from the 2005 and 2006 HealthStyles survey. *Public Health Rep*. (1974) 2011;126 (Suppl 1):100–107.

Klein-Schwartz W, Oderda GM. Poisoning in the elderly. Epidemiological, clinical and management considerations. *Drugs Aging*. 1991;Jan 1;1(1): 67–89.

Medeiros-Sousa P, dos Santos-Neto L, Kusano L, Pereira M. Diagnosis and control of polypharmacy in the elderly. *Rev Saude Publica*. 2007;41(6): 1049–53.

Merck Manuals Online Medical Library on Poisoning: merck.com/mmhe /sec24/ch297/ch297a.html.

Non-fatal, unintentional, non-fire-related carbon monoxide exposures. United States, 2004–2006. *MMWR Morb Mortal Wkly Rep*. 2008;Aug. 22; 57(33):896-99.

Poisoning in the United States: Fact Sheet: cdc.gov/homeandrecreational safety/poisoning/poisoning-factsheet.htm.

Schiffman SS. Taste and smell losses in normal aging and disease. *JAMA*. 1997;Oct. 22–29;278(16):1357–62.

Smith JL. Foodborne illness in the elderly. *J Food Prot*. 1998;Sep.;61(9):1229–39.

State laws concerning carbon monoxide: ncsl.org/default.aspx?tabid =13238#tx.

Tyk C. Prevention of medication error and unintentional drug poisoning in the elderly. Editorial. *Hong Kong Med J*. 2006;Oct.;12(no. 5):332–33.

UPI International. Many unaware of N.Y. CO detector law. *Health News*, Mar. 2, 2011. upi.com/Health_News/2011/03/02/Many-unaware-of-NY -CO-detector-law/UPI-67101299123116/#ixzz1G1kGue93.

Vann M. Is your food still safe to eat? At everydayhealth.com/digestive
-health/how-long-is-my-food-safe-to-eat.aspx.

Chapter 5. Preventing Asphyxia

Chillag S, Krieg J, Bhargava R. The Heimlich maneuver: breaking down the
complications. *South Med J*. 2010;Feb.;103(2):147–50.
Dolkas L, Stanley C, Smith AM, Vilke GM. Deaths associated with choking
in San Diego County. *J Forensic Sci*. 2007;Jan.;52(1):176–79.
Food and Drug Administration, Center for Devices and Radiologic Health.
Hospital bed dimensional and assessment guidance to reduce entrap-
ment. Mar. 10, 2006. www.fda.gov/MedicalDevices/DeviceRegulation
andGuidance/GuidanceDocuments/ucm072662.htm#8.
National Safety Council choking information: nsc.org/SAFETY_HOME
/HOMEANDRECREATIONALSAFETY/Pages/Choking.aspx.
Preventing suffocation and choking injuries in Manitoba: a review of best
practices. 2006. Injury Prevention Centre of Children's Hospital.
gov.mb.ca/healthyliving/hlp/docs/injury/injuries_suffocation.pdf.
Roy N, Stemple J, Merrill RM, Thomas L. Dysphagia in the elderly: prelim-
inary evidence of prevalence, risk factors, and socioemotional effects.
Ann Otol Rhinol Laryngol. 2007;Nov.;116(11):858–65.

Chapter 6. When Driving Is Dangerous

Adler G. Driving decision-making in older adults with dementia. *Dementia*
(Sage). 2010;9(1):45–60.
Bauzá G, Lamorte WW, Burke PA, Hirsch EF. High mortality in elderly
drivers is associated with distinct injury patterns: analysis of 187,869
injured drivers. *J Trauma*. 2008;Feb.;64(2):304–10.
Carr DB, Ott BR. The older adult driver with cognitive impairment: "It's a
very frustrating life." *JAMA*. 2010;303(16):1632–41.
Deladisma AM, Parker W, Medeiros R, Hawkins ML. All-terrain vehicle
trauma in the elderly: an analysis of a national database. *Am Surg*. 2008;
74(8):767–69.
Donorfio LK, D'Ambrosio LA, Coughlin JF, Mohyde M. Health, safety, self-
regulation and the older driver: It's not just a matter of age. *J Safety Res*.
2008;39(6):555–61.
Donorfio LK, D'Ambrosio LA, Coughlin JF, Mohyde M. To drive or not to
drive, that isn't the question—the meaning of self-regulation among
older drivers. *J Safety Res*. 2009;40(3):221–26.

Gentzler MD, Smither JA. A literature review of major perceptual, cognitive, and/or physical test batteries for older drivers. *Work*. 2012;41:5381–83.

Horswill MS, Anstey KJ, Hatherly C, Wood JM, Pachana NA. Older drivers' insight into their hazard perception ability. *Accid Anal Prev*. 2011;43(6): 2121–27.

Hu G, Baker SP. Recent increases in fatal and non-fatal injury among people aged 65 years and over in the USA. *Injury Prevention*. 2010;16:26–30.

Hunt LA, Brown AE, Gilman IP. Drivers with dementia and outcomes of becoming lost while driving. *Am J Occup Ther*. 2010;64(2):225–32.

Kay LG, Bundy A, Clemson L. Validity, reliability and predictive accuracy of the Driving Awareness Questionnaire. *Disabil Rehabil*. 2009;31(13): 1074–82.

Lavallière M, Laurendeau D, Simoneau M, Teasdale N. Changing lanes in a simulator: effects of aging on the control of the vehicle and visual inspection of mirrors and blind spot. *Traffic Injury Prev*. 2011;12(2):191–200.

National Highway Transportation Safety Administration. Occupant protection issues among older drivers and passengers: volume 1. Final Report. DOT HS 810 938. Apr. 2008.

O'Connor MG, Kapust LR, Hollis AM. DriveWise: an interdisciplinary hospital-based driving assessment program. *Gerontol Geriatr Educ*. 2008; 29(4):351–62.

Thompson KR, Johnson AM, Emerson JL, Dawson JD, Boer ER, Rizzo M. Distracted driving in elderly and middle-aged drivers. *Accid Anal Prev*. 2012;45(2):711–17.

Van Ranst E, Silverstein NM, Gottlieb AS. Promoting safe and comfortable driving for elders. In *Future of Intelligent and Extellingent Health Environment*. Edited by RG Bushko. Amsterdam: IOS Press; 2005.

Van Roosmalen L, Paquin GJ, Steinfeld AM. Quality of life technology: the state of personal transportation. *Phys Med Rehabil Clin N Am*. 2010;21(1): 111–25.

Vardaki S, Yannis G. Investigation of the acceptance of a handbook for safe driving at an older age. *Int J Inj Control Safe Promot*. 2012;19(1):27–36.

Wang CC, Carr DB. Older driver safety: a report from the Older Drivers Project. *J Amer Geriatrics Soc*. 2004;Jan.;52(1):143–49. DOI: 10.1111/j. 1532-5415.2004.52025.x.

Young MS, Bunce D. Driving into the sunset: supporting cognitive functioning in older drivers. *J Aging Res*. 2011; Article ID 918782, 6 pages; DOI 10.4061/2011/918782.

Chapter 7. The Backyard and the Workshop

American Lyme Disease Foundation, Inc., P.O. Box 466, Lyme, CT 06371; http://www.aldf.com/lyme.shtml.

American National Standards Institute, Inc. ANSI A14.2 Ladders—Portable Metal—Safety Requirements. DesPlaines; American Society of Safety Engineers; 1990.

Deladisma AM, Parker W, Medeiros R, Hawkins ML. All-terrain vehicle trauma in the elderly: an analysis of a national database. *Am Surg.* 2008; 74(8):767–69.

Hammig B, Jones C. Injuries related to snow blowers in the United States, 2002 through 2008. *Acad Emerg Med.* 2010;17(5):566-69. DOI 10.1111/j.1553-2712.2010.00730.x.

Lyme disease information: ncbi.nlm.nih.gov/pubmedhealth/PMH000 2296/.

Poisonous plants information: www.cdc.gov/niosh/topics/plants/.

Rutherford, GD. Baby boomer sports injuries. *Inj Control Safe Promo.* 2001; 8(1):51–53.

US Consumer Product Safety Commission. Fiscal 2013 operating plan; www.cpsc.gov/library/foia/foia13/brief/2013operatingplan.pdf.

US Consumer Product Safety Commission. Table saw blade contact injuries; Advance notice of proposed rulemaking; Request for comments and information; www.cpsc.gov/BUSINFO/frnotices/fr12/tablesaw ANPR.pdf.

Chapter 8. All around the House

Home safety for people with Alzheimer's disease. NIH Publication 02-5179. Bethesda, MD: National Institute on Aging; Dec. 2008.

Mertens B, Sorenson SB. Current considerations about the elderly and firearms. *Amer J Pub Health.* 2012;102(3):396–400.

Telecoil information: www.nchearingloss.org/telecoil.htm?fromncshhh.

Chapter 9. Seeing the Doctor

Ahluwalia K. Oral healthcare for the elderly: more than just dentures. *Am J Public Health.* 2004;May 94(5):698;ncbi.nlm.nih.gov/pmc/articles/PMC 1448318/pdf/0940698.pdf.

American Academy of Audiology. www.audiology.org/Pages/default.aspx.

American Speech-Language-Hearing Association. www.asha.org.

Ask Me 3. National Patient Safety Foundation. www.npsf.org/askme3.

Bostock S, Steptoe A. Association between low functional health literacy and mortality in older adults: longitudinal cohort study. *BMJ.* 2012;Mar. 15;344:e1602. DOI: 10.1136/bmj.e1602.

Federal Trade Commission advice on hearing aids: ftc.gov/bcp/edu/pubs /consumer/health/hea10.shtml. See also ftc.gov/whocares.

Food and Drug Administration advice on hearing aids: fda.gov/Medical Devices/ProductsandMedicalProcedures/HomeHealthandConsumer /ConsumerProducts/HearingAids/default.htm.

McCarthy DM, Waite KR, Curtis LM, Engel KG, Baker DW, Wolf MS. What did the doctor say? Health literacy and recall of medical instructions. *Care.* 2012;Apr.;50(4):277–82.

MedlinePlus. www.nlm.nih.gov/medlineplus.

National Institute on Deafness and Other Communication Disorders www.nidcd.nih.gov.

Old Colony Memorial. May 30, 2012; ID: 12bf475985edec803d75a2cf6295ddlc.

Talking with your doctor: a guide for older people. NIH Publication 05-3452. Bethesda, MD: National Institute on Aging; 2005; reprinted Apr. 2008.

INDEX